ABO PLUS

THE FINAL DIET

By

Marcello Menapace, PhD, MChem, MBA

ABO PLUS

THE FINAL DIET

By

Marcello Menapace, PhD, MChem, MBA

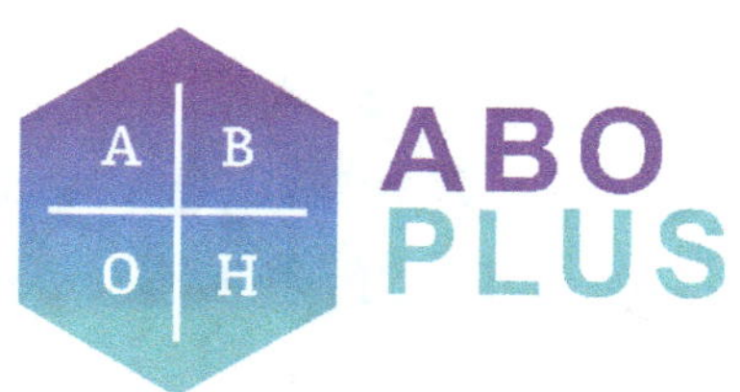

Registered Trademark

Copyright

Illustrations by

Salvatore "Turi" Papale

www.turipapale.com

General Curator and Book Cover Design

Dr. Maria Ferrara

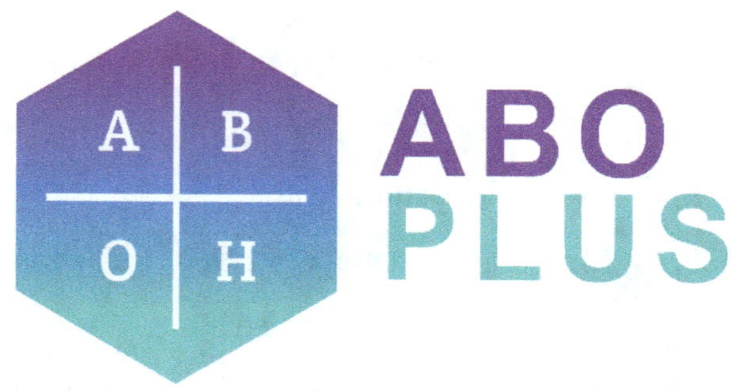

ABO PLUS is a Registered Trademark

Registration UK00003804373

Table of Contents

Table of Contents

p. 1/193

Foreword

This is a very straightforward book for the understanding the ABO-PLUS™ method (the ultimate lifestyle and diet method). In this book, you will learn about the re-discovery of ancient medicine in its pure western (Graeco-Roman) form and its inclusion into the overall health system defined as ABO-PLUS™. Essentially, ABO-PLUS™ is the fusion of the blood type diet, as demonstrated scientifically by the author Dr Marcello Menapace, and the Western form of ancient medicine in a truly holistic and personalized medical system that everybody can learn.

What I call Western Constitutional Medicine (WCM), is intuitively easy to grasp. One of the most important achievements of the so-called Greek-Roman medicine (WCM), was the concept of biotypology (in other terms constitution, or body make).

We, humans, are not just plain human beings being composed only of human cells, which are occasionally attacked by viruses and bacteria generating diseases. No. This is an incorrect and incomplete concept. We are "holobionts". We are a balanced mix of all forms of life, from unicellular to pluricellular organisms. These bugs are living together and are integrated into what can be called a "human being". All ancient medicines (including WCM) embraced the idea of equilibrium (as way of reasoning) between forms of life living within us. The practitioners of TCAMs proposed as a remedy the return to the original state of equilibrium. To do this, the main strategy adopted by all medicinal systems in the past was dietary intervention. The famous phrase by the father of Medicine, Hippocrates, "let food be thy medicine and medicine be thy food" is a testament to this. Diet is thus a good method for the correction of disharmonious states and for the restoration of the equilibrium between the energies (bugs) in the body. More recently though another type of new medicinal system, the ABO blood type diet was established. This diet or system has become ever more important in the scientific world. As experimental confirmation of its main mechanism of action became evident, we could not forsake this new diet. Many new technical fields related to the sciences of carbohydrates (especially glycobiology) proved its mechanism of action and transformed ABO blood type diet into a reality. All bugs eat small carbohydrates (glycans) in a differential manner. So, ABO glycans are connected to different bugs in the human body. And this also explains its action.

Inevitably, microscopic bugs (bacteria), fungi and other unicellular organisms have been shown to feed off on glycans which are both produced (ABO and others) and absorbed (diet) by the human body and the suitable balance of diet will interfere in this cycle. Time has come to secure all these advances in knowledge from ancient and modern medicine and combine them into a new medicinal system, ABO PLUS™. ABO PLUS™, that is the ABO-WCM biotypology, can factually better explain the reality of the holobiont and completely transform modern science into a truly personalized approach.

The healing interventions proposed by ABO PLUS™ are based on nutritional (i.e., what they should tendentially eat and drink) and physical therapies depending on their constitution with the use of natural (vitamins and minerals) and herbal products.

As a disclaimer, please note also that this book is a starter guide and cannot explain all the complexities of the therapeutic potential of the ABO-PLUS™ method nor its actual application. However, it can give you a lot of suggestions and interesting information about your body and mind. Only a skilled expert can adapt this method to your personal needs and any real-world health issues.

1 Introduction

We all hear continuously in TV, radio, and journals technical terms like "Molecular Nutrition" or "biochemical reaction" and what not concerning diets. Although these complex terms are not meant to scare off the audience but to discuss on precise terminologies, it has the unwanted effect to put down the non-experts in the field. This is too bad because we all need to understand the world in which we live in and to take advantage of the accumulated evidence in science on how to make our own lives better. Thus, this book is also about how to maintain health and reach certain objectives one has in mind.

As mentioned before (foreword), this book is essentially a starter guide and cannot explain all the complexities of the therapeutic potential of the ABO-PLUS™ method, but it can give you a lot of tips and interesting information about your body and mind.

We have all been sick at least once in our lifetime. For many people this occurs more often than what we would like it to be. And even more often illness just happens perchance, without us knowing why.

We are told by many doctors (clinicians, general practitioners, and physicians), as the experts of a branch of science called medicine, that it just happens to be so that someone gets ill and there's almost no way to prevent it. Sure, the health community does like to repeat that one must try to embrace a healthy lifestyle (eat healthy and exercise daily), but when it comes to practical advice, the communication is broken down. Any kind of dietary recommendation is way too general and not specific to everyone's conditions or genetic make-up.

1.1 Different People

This is the central theme of the book: general advice more often results useless.

The premise at the base of most diets and therapeutic systems is that we are all humans thus we will react similarly to the same interventions.

This is a big presupposition. And we need to really dot the i's and cross the t's.

If we look at the big picture, we will find that, as humans, we will react in a similar way but biologically it will be slightly different. An example: if we cut ourselves (like a papercut), some people will bleed abundantly (just like me) some will not. Some people will heal quickly some will not. Some people will not feel any pain, some will feel a lot more.

As you can notice, people necessarily react differently. Not just physiologically or biologically but also psychologically. These factors have to be taken into consideration in any method to understand and attempt to alleviate the health issues of people. Being distinct and unique, we will need to look into the reasons for this difference between people. Once we have learned about this, we can see how extensive these are.

But we are lucky. This has already been done.

No, not by myself. Much, much earlier.

I am just putting together what was known for millennia on the one hand and what has been discovered in the past century.

For the very first time, a new system, ABO PLUS™, has been devised. This system explains why different people obtain different results using the same diets or exercises, etc. It uses the two major systems that classify humans in various distinct groups physically and biochemically.

In this new system, you will find the answers to your most compelling questions, such as: "Why can't I achieve my goals as other people do?" Or "Why am I eating as much as any other individual or even less, but I don't lose weight?" Or "Why am I exercising so much but my muscles do not grow enough as I would like to?"

Not that you have to lose weight. Only if this is your goal. In any case, it becomes stressful.

It's frustrating. More than that, even. Most of the times it makes you feel "sad", "gloomy" and "depressed". I bet it is a terrible feeling. I know, in one way or the other we have all gone through such experiences that we would have never wished to go through. And after that what happens? Well, we lose all our resolve and surrender to the bleak reality. Then we tend to go back to our previous habits, losing all the small successes we have achieved.

This happens also with health. We eat what we think it's healthy but then we do not see any improvement. And sometimes our symptoms even get worse.

The problem with all the other diets and strategies that we have been trying for all these years is that they are missing a fundamental point. We are unique, each single one of us. No one is identical to another person. Not even homozygous twins. Not morphologically (meaning physically), nor biochemically.

Look, we just need to realize that what a person can do easily, another would take a lot of effort. And we have all experienced something like that. Certain people are naturally driven towards singing, others towards drawing, others towards driving cars, etc. The list is almost limitless. The point that needs to be made is that there are specific differences that makes us unique, special and simply beautiful.

The big mistake for most diets and medical systems is to say that any therapy or intervention will always give the same result. This is absurd, to say the least. And we experience this every day. People eat the same food and some experience nothing, others feel bloated, others still have an immune or allergic reaction, etc. And sometimes this is on a scale with several degrees of severity, depending on your genetic make-up.

We all know that this makes us feel bad, and often we feel guilty. We tend to put the blame on us or on our weak will while the culprit is somewhere else, most of the time.

The missing point with all other diets and therapies is this: they do not put together the two foundational characteristics of our body: its structure (body shape or biotype) and ABO blood type. These two dissimilar factors, which belong to the genetics of our own human body (physical for the biotype and biochemical for the ABO blood type), define who we are. Not just that, these two attributes make us biochemically and physically different from others. But within certain limits.

1.2   Blood Type Diet

So, what is the reason then for another book on the Blood Type Diet (BTD)?

It's not. It is a book regarding ABO-PLUS. The new system that literally puts together two approaches to our different body characteristics.

First, the explanation ever given in favor of BTDs is incomplete, at best. Indeed, we have been told that special proteins in foods (called "lectins") can bind to carbohydrates on the surface of human cells (called "glycans") and thus cause reactions (simplified explanation). While this is true, it is not the whole story! Only when we take into consideration all the molecules in foods and on the cell surfaces ("membranes"), we can better understand what is going on.

Secondly, only understanding the true biochemical pathways and explaining them without hard words allow non-experts in nutrition to learn the dietary tricks that can be used in their personal eating patterns.

Thirdly, once the key to open the lock is understood, everything else becomes plain and straightforward. It is neither difficult nor complex to comprehend once it is explained in non-technical words. Moreover, the method can be used every time you need it.

We are all different and individually unique, even if we all belong to the same human family. Our skin may have different shades of color and so our eyes and hair are colored slightly differently among us. We are tall or short, thin, or bulky and stronger or weaker: all different in our one matchless characteristic. Undeniably, I am stating the obvious here!

Due to our uniqueness, each person is slightly dissimilar in several ways (at least, physically but also biochemically). Notwithstanding this, we are all identical morally and intellectually (as human beings, males, and females alike). These little alterations are what makes us exceptional and rare. No two human beings are identical and indistinguishable in every way.

Perhaps the most important external agent that affects us all is food. For example, we all know by experience that some people simply cannot tolerate eating certain food items or feel sick when eating others. These effects and symptoms (commonly called "clinical manifestations") highlight the fact that there is some form of intolerance or sensitivity, demonstrating that we are all different and distinct. Even in the Bible, as a text written thousands of years ago, this fact was well known.

Again, one of the most clear-cut differences between each one of us is our blood type. This is of course the main focus of this small guide: the ABO blood groups define our intimate characteristics and then explain how food reacts differentially to the various blood groups. We all should be familiar with the fact that everyone has one and only one blood type: either A, B, O or AB. True, there are a few individuals in the world that are neither (H-), but these people are extremely rare there are not enough available study to draw any rational conclusions on their dietary patterns.

It should not be a surprise that the biochemical difference imposed by the blood type we have (technically called "ABO typology"), unique to each person, factually distinguishes us based on the way we react to chemical compounds present in foods. From this we can conclude that each person has its own personal intolerances and ways in which we become sick ("disease susceptibilities").

I have given you here a very compressed explanation of how the blood type affects our responses to food with simple and complex words (identified by "biochemical interactions"). This could be sufficient for you to have a rough idea on how things truly work. But I would be a liar to state that this is it. I would like to go in a bit more detail in the next Chapter to show you how things operate at the smaller ("molecular") level. I assure you it will not be complex or tedious to appreciate.

I would like to stress on the concept of health and disease by making clear that there truly IS such a thing like a division between general advice for a group of individuals (belonging to a specific blood type) and specific advice for each individual person (as previously hinted to). The way we now understand health and disease and I present it here in this mini guide may differ from that generally taught and marketed by standard medicine ("biomedicine"). Modern medicine is more interested in how to make you feel better (i.e., the treatment of diseases) by helping you cope with the symptoms ("symptomatic treatment") and not much in the understanding of the causes of diseases. This is separate with what I share with you in this book. Once we identify the causes of most diseases, it will be easier for us to avoid the consequences of diseases (i.e., their symptoms) by simply removing, where possible, those causes. Of course, I do not perform miracles!

Now, the major causes can be explained through the recourse to molecular Nutrition. It is inevitable that many topics will cross into the domain of medicine and other fields of science. Hence it is important to clarify from the beginning which concepts will be taken from medicine and which from each of the several scientific fields of study.

All this will be accomplished without recurring to unproven concepts and theories. We shall remain most attached to physical reality and to what we can see, hear, smell, taste, touch and prove by repeatable experiments, the ones you and I can do in the kitchen.

Before we start in this short journey to understand health as linked to what we eat (nutrition), I would like to clarify what I mean with blood type. When you go to the doctor (a physician/ clinician like your general practitioner or your family doctor) and ask her/ him, what is your blood type (should you not know), she/ he will tell you that you are either A or B or O or AB and positive or negative. The A or B or O or AB identifies the main characteristic of your blood: these are the names of small carbohydrate molecules present on the cells of your blood (the "red blood cells", the ones that transport oxygen). These small carbohydrates are commonly grouped together and abbreviated as ABO. The positive or negative instead identifies a very important protein present on those same cells called Rhesus factor (thus you will hear the term Rhesus type positive or negative). We will focus on the carbohydrates as these are the main

Although the term "carbohydrate" points to the molecules constituting bread, pizza, or pasta the same expression is used to generically identify all the plethora of molecules (small and large alike) that have some basic common features resembling those of sugar. You might have heard in school talking about the following words: proteins, fat, and nucleic acids. These are three of the four main (and only) big and abundant (that's the reason why they are termed "macro") molecules constituting us and our food.

While I don't want to get into the nighty gritty of the distinctions between these macromolecules (big and abundant in our body), I do want to emphasize on carbohydrates and their shape and form. No, don't worry, I will not go into the chemical definitions and structures of them but, like an architect that shows a model of your house before they proceed with the building and restauration, I do want to show you the model of these molecules.

If you are healthy, it is really your choice to try this nutritional approach. If you do not have any symptoms, you can even decide to give it a try (as a sort of detoxification) for a week or a month, based on the effects of this diet on your body. If you have severe diseases (e.g., autoimmune diseases), you might want to discuss about this diet with your doctor, since it might be beneficial for you. You can also follow these suggestions during the week and have a cheating day where you eat whatever you please. It is up to you and your body's responses and your energy level.

With no further ado, let's jump right into the preparatory part of this mini-Guide.

2 Traditional Medicine

Let's face the bare facts: medicine is not a science. You can call it whatever you would like, and it is fine. Science is one thing and medicine is another. It may be based on science, sure. But they're not the same.

Science is experimentation with repeatable results. Not so medicine. Why? Because, one thing stands out, among them all: we, human beings, are all different. And being different, we respond differently to different diseases and therapies.

No one single therapy or therapeutic option is valid or useful for every single individual present on this Earth.

Medicine is a profession, an art with masters and a practice, from whence we get the name 'practitioners'. So, similarly to law or other practices, medicine requires a person to enter into an official registry. Although it is loosely based on science, medicine is the experience of a practitioner in learning how to deal with people and with their health problems. I say loosely because it is practiced against a background of incomplete scientific knowledge about the nature of disease processes.

It goes without saying that modern allopathic system of medicine (what we call biomedicine, or simply contemporary medicine) has made great strides and contribution to the understanding of human physiology and cellular metabolic pathways. It has also brought out very effective methodologies for handling short term and emergency health conditions, such as acute diseases and infections. But there is a problem with long, time-consuming, chronic diseases which have no resolutive treatment with modern allopathic medicine.

The specialization trend in medicine is certainly one of the most common problems we see today. You see patients being thrown literally from one specialist to the other often without any success in finding the correct treatment for an unknown disease. Specialization means essentially looking at an elephant with a magnifying glass: the best thing you could find is some bugs if you're lucky, but you won't find the elephant itself. It is not possible to see the big picture (the overall cause of a health state) with all these super-detailed analysis and sectorial way of thinking.

It is time to look somewhere else to see what they have to say.

2.1 Early history of western medicine

Initially, early medicine was practiced in the form of preventive medicine as in the times of ancient Egypt through to the Babylonian civilization. And surely though gradually a body of knowledge based on chance observation and trial and error was accumulating. Then, came the time of Hippocrates (c. 400 BC), the first true western physician and surgeon, the greatest of ancient Greece.

But the ancient people were no stupid humans. They were extremely gifted, smart, and clever, much more than we are now. Just look at the mummification process of ancient Egyptians, with the removal of most of the internal organs including the brain, lungs, pancreas, liver, spleen, heart, and intestine. Or look at the trephination (or trepanning of the skull) process recovered in prehistoric tombs and written down in the Hammurabi code, where the eye and brain surgeons would pay a dear price, by law, if they were to make a mistake. And many other countless techniques used in the past that we just recently became familiar with.

Anyway, the medical knowledge derived from the ancients forms the basis of our current practice of medicine today. The great expertise acquired by the Egyptians was then transferred on to the Greeks and to the Romans.

By the beginning of the first millennium AD, three main systems of medicine were available: Ayurveda, Greek and Chinese medicine; and the Greek have taken advantage of the unparalleled experience of the Egyptians. Egyptian medicine was so advanced that they were able to describe the anatomy and physiology of the body and tumors, due to corpse dissection, only surpassed by twentieth century medicine.

2.2 Alternatives

Conventional (modern) medicine has become too dependent on very expensive technological solutions to health problems, even when they are not particularly effective. This is obviously not available in poor countries.

Because, as said before, the expansion of Western medicine is limited, in the 1980s traditional systems of medicine (CAMs) contributed significantly to the medical needs of 80% of the world's population. Even more, traditional medicine (TM) in the East has been integrated with official westernized medicine so that

India, China, Korea, Taiwan, and Japan have all national health systems which offer both alternatives.

Most recently, by the start of the 21st century, a medical perspective emerged (constitutional medicine) based on a holistic view of the organism. This new (really?) concept rejected the approaches of microbiology and modern allopathic medicine. The idea of alternative medicine is based on the primacy of clinical medicine (what the doctors can see for themselves) and proposed an individualized/personalized conception of illnesses (holistic).

Among the long list of therapies, which includes necessarily traditional Chinese medicine (TCM), available in the world, it would be interesting to focus momentarily on two ancient medicinal systems.

1. Unani (Tibb)

Unani Tibb (Ionian/Greek medicine in Arabic) is one of the ancient systems of medicine still used today in South Asia and the Middle East. It forms an integral part of national healthcare system in India. Unani medicine refers to a tradition of Greek-Arabic medicine which is based on the teachings of Greek physician Buqrat (Hippocrates), Roman physician Jalinoos (Galen) and developed by Arab and Persian physicians such as Al Razi (Rhazes), Ibn sina (Avicenna), Al Zahrawi and Ibn Nafis.

So, it is essentially a flavor of western constitution medicine. We would say an Arabic twist of WCM.

2. Tibetan Medicine

Tibetan medicine was developed thousands of years ago and utilized the ancient concept of three humors. While WCM used four and TCM five, Tibetan medicine is more similar to the three ayurvedic Doshas. As we will see, a tradition of medicine using a specific number of humors is always valid within that system.

The individual's humoral constitution in Tibetan medicine can be determined as early as infancy (being modulated by the diet and behavior of a child's mother during pregnancy) and is regulated by the three humors: rlung (wind), mkhris pa (fire), and bad kan (earth and water).

Further CAMs could be listed and detailed but it is preferable to focus on the scientific basis through which all these operate.

2.3   Constitutional Medicine or Biotypology

All traditional forms of medicine, especially all ancient traditions in the east, use the concept of constitutions. A constitution is linked to the prevailing humor present in the human body of that specific person. Thus, in a system of medicine entailing three humors, at least 3 different types of individuals can be identified by a practitioner. If a system has four humors, then four types of persons can be classified. And so on, so forth.

The constitution is roughly defined as a predetermined mixture of certain characteristics and features, such as body mass, strength, etc. In other words, it is an integrated, relatively stable state of morphological, physiological, and psychological attributes based on genetic and acquired factors.

These groups of persons having similar physical and/or biochemical characteristics belong to a class called biotype. A biotype or somatotype is a type of person with similar physical or biochemical features.

The medicine that evaluates, defines and/or uses the biotype idea is called constitutional medicine. The study of biotypes is named biotypology.

Biotypology is used to identify the main constitutional type of each patient. Once this is done, the practitioner will then discover their innate tendency to manifest certain symptoms and diseases. These properties belong to the biotype. And each biotype has different features, leading to specific patterns in predisposition to particular pathologies (diseases).

The age-old Latin adage, developed by the Romans, '*mens sana in corpore sano*' (loosely translated as: a healthy mind is in a healthy body) not only summarizes the essence of all traditional medicinal systems but also does convey this message of superior harmony between the mind and the body.

As humans are extremely intricate, to adequately conceptualize a person in health or illness requires an approach that is not reducible into thousands of subfield, as is done in modern medicine. Traditional medicinal systems have the capacity to leverage such a vast complexity by adopting multidimensional and multidirectional models (biotypology and personalization).

At the present stage of the medical development, the treatment of disease should be achieved with a combination of the modern classical methods developed by medical science and with the complementary use of the most effective methods of 'traditional' medicine. Integrative medicine — i.e., combining traditional and folk knowledge —is the medicine of the future. It is the idea of integrating the old with the new that can finally provide us with new methods for diagnosis and allow treatment to be maximally effective.

2.4 Conclusions

Modern medicine has traveled a long path since the time of Hippocrates and has gained an enormous amount of specialized knowledge. But with all this knowledge, modern medicine is losing sight with the wholeness (holistic approach) of the human body.

Hippocrates has laid the foundations of the modern theory that thoughts, ideas and feelings can influence health and the process of disease. He attributed diseases to natural causes, believed in the healing power of nature, and gave special emphasis to the prevention and prognosis (prediction of the course) of illnesses. He treated patients as psychosomatic entities (a holistic medical approach) in relation to their natural environment.

p. 19/193

The same thing happened and still happens with those Eastern traditional medicines that are actively practiced today in many World regions. They are founded on the concept of constitution (body type) and all remedies are focused on bringing back harmony in that specific biotype.

So too is ancient western medicine (WCM). Being based on biotypology and the differences between people belonging to various classified groups, WCM could adopt the right treatments for all people. And this allowed WCM to reach incredibly successful results.

Modern scientific materialism (or the reductionist worldview where all is just matter) is way too out of hand with this reality. Although this is the leading ideological belief system in modern society, it is incorrect. It has unjustly dominated world thought from the late nineteenth century and early twentieth century. We must try to stand clear from this nonsense and just look at the bare facts: if a method works, then it's good, whatever the mechanism of action.

Thus, we should highlight what is advantageous and experimentally sound in any area. If the theory around biotypes is sound and prove then we should embrace it, regardless of its origin or of our political ideals, or philosophical stance or even religious nature.

Finally, ancient medicine recognized that we all are different, but also comparable (alike) within particular parameters. Ancient medicine acknowledged the differences and similarities and defined these in classification systems known as biotypologies. These ancient systems of classification allowed practitioners to better understand each individual physical and physiological uniqueness. They uncovered our limits and potentialities enclosed in our bodies and used them to devise remedies that were appropriate for each person (tailored therapies).

p. 20/193

3 The Biological Explanation

<u>Disclaimer</u>

This chapter is about how the ABO-PLUS™ system and diet actually works. It is a scientific explanation, even though with simple and understandable words and concepts. It is not essential, so if you don't want to know how it works, just jump this whole chapter and go to the next. There is no need to read this if you don't want to, but you might discover interesting facts if you give it a try.

3.1 Introduction

The first fact that will shock you is this: we've all got bugs!

And when I say all, I really mean "all people": every single person on the face of the Earth, that has ever lived or ever will live, at any single point in time of their existence. No exceptions.

And what do I mean with "bugs"? I mean microorganisms (microbes). Anything that is living but very, very little. From bacteria, to protozoa, to fungi to viruses. Anything of this sort, we have them all in our body.

Now you could say: "Oh, no. This is gross!". Go on, say that. But this won't change the fact that we have them. At least, this much science has confirmed incontrovertibly in the last 20 years.

The human body during health and disease states, alike, contains many different places (or habitats) that are occupied by microbes. And the number and type of these microbial populations differ considerably from person to person. To be clear, if each of us had available a list of species of bugs (types of microbes) and relative amounts, and were we to compare them, these would be all different. Full stop!

These microbiological (bacteriological and more) communities, termed "microbiota" (a fancy name for living microbes residing somewhere in us) is made up of several predominant bacterial phyla (composed of literally hundreds, if not thousands, of bacterial species and genera).

And now the second fact that will likely startle you: as a whole, the microbiota outnumbers human cells in the body by an estimated two to one! That is, if we have 1 trillion cells in our body, the number of bacterial and fungal cell would equate to 2 trillion. Pretty stunning!

But how did we get to know all these things and much more? By the use of novel techniques of gene sequencing called 16S ribosomal gene-specific next generation sequencing (NGS). But I won't bother you with such details.

The fact of the matter is this: we have been able to find microbial genetic material (DNA and/or RNA), in places we previously thought were sterile in the human body.

The use of these next-gen technologies has allowed us to realize that we were wrong in considering the human body as essentially aseptic (sterile). We are quickly realizing that many bacterial and viral species, which are successfully fitted to the human body, cannot not be cultured (or identified via an old technique to grow bugs), at all. It was only through the development of these technologies that we discovered this.

An analysis of 27 different body sites, including the skin, nostril, hair, brain, heart, and oral cavity revealed that distinctive anatomical niches exist and are the homeplace to unique microbes. Unique means preferentially living in that habitat.

This is not just amazing, we are thunderstruck: it seems to be unbelievable, but true.

3.2 Human Body Habitats

Now we all knew, or must have known by now, that the gastrointestinal tract (GIT), is home to the most abundant microbial community in the entire human body. It has been known for several decades to harbor microbial colonies. This delicate and balanced ecosystem in the human intestine, in which 10 to the power of 14 (that is a number with 14 zeros behind it) bacteria dwell routinely and prosper, forms the human gut "microflora" (another word for microbiota).

It has now been established that the living bacteria in the intestines are helpful to the human body in several ways. It seems that the establishment of an equilibrium between tissue and microbes is a fundamental concept that underlines all human-microbe interactions. As for gut microbiota, this result introduced the concept of <u>tissue-microbe equilibrium,</u> as a potential factor in human health.

Several tissues and human body regions are commonly colonized by live bacteria, healthily dwelling, and providing support for us as humans (see Figure 1). We find them on the skin, in the lungs and generally along the airways, in the urinary system and in the stomach, just to name a few.

Figure 1. A few regions shown to be harboring non-human life

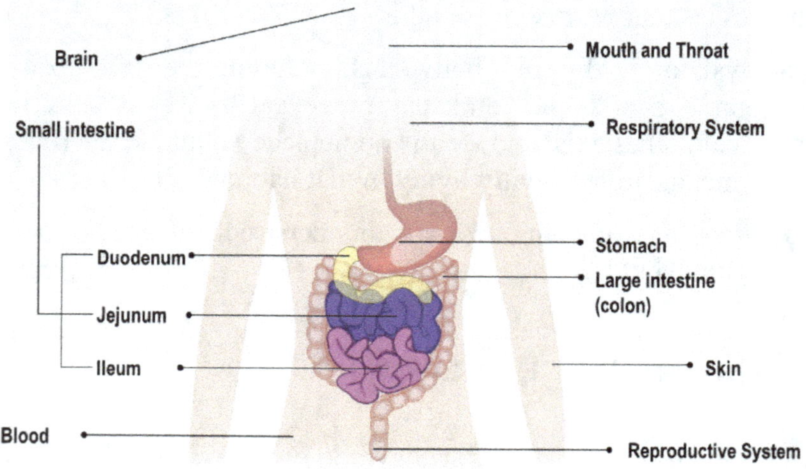

Places where we have found microbes living happily with us.

Perhaps the most extraordinary thing that occurred in the last 20 odd years in science is the realization that microbes are normally in the blood, previously thought to be absolutely sterile. Remarkably, the human blood of healthy individuals is not believed anymore to be sterile, but to contain its own microbiome (as community of microbes.

Conversely, other microbes that are not "endemic" or commensal to that habitat but are nevertheless found there are pathogenic (noxious). Their presence may very well disrupt the normal co-living conditions of other microbes generating a disease.

p. 24/193

Up until recently, intrauterine infection of the placenta was thought to be the cause of several fetal diseases. But more recent studies have shown that the human placenta is colonized not only by bacteria, but also that this placental microbial community exists has a unique composition which resembles that of an oral microbiota.

The composition of these microbial communities is specific for each tissue and adapted to it so that they live in symbiosis (i.e., helping the host and receiving nourishment from the host). Whenever a different typology of bacterial species establishes itself in a particular habitat, where it is not endemic, something bad happens. In these events, these foreign microorganisms become necessarily pathogenic (that is dangerous) as they reduce the space occupied by the resident species and therefore the amount of positive biochemical feedback that commensal microbes provide. These events, in the end, create a state of disequilibrium (dysbiosis) in the tissue where the event occurred, and this is the hallmark of disease.

All these studies demonstrate continually that microbes may well be resident in all tissues in healthy conditions as symbionts but when an undesired condition occurs, a change in the preexisting equilibrium (from eubiosis to dysbiosis) brings about a state od disease.

3.3 The Holobiont

3.3.1 The notion

There is a brand-new idea that has been silently gaining ground as of late that promises to transform for good the way we think about biology, forever. This novel idea is the result of the realization of the human body as a mixture of different species of cells. The concept is called the holobiont: the host and its associated microorganisms which form communities within the body.

This new notion of the holobiont is like the idea of a new "self": a real change in the way we should think of ourselves. The novel view is that we, humans, are truly a dynamic, balanced, and interactive community (seen as a collection) of human and microbial cells. To be more transparent and clear-cut: We, as humans, could be considered as hybrid organisms, consisting of both human (eukaryotic) and bacterial (prokaryotic) cells.

Humans are thus holobionts and as such have special and unthought of before qualities. A holobiont is thus an individual with an emergent phenotype (external characteristics) composed of both his or her own genome and the vast resident microbiota's genetic material.

The health of the holobiont (the microbe-host system), relies on a wide-range of biochemical or physical interactions between the host and its resident bugs. The immune system has been the first human physiologic system to be linked with the two-way regulation of and by the gut resident bacteria. The microbiota has been implicated in:

1. the modulation of the gut-brain axis (alteration of behavior and regulation of central nervous system molecular changes;

2. The production of neurotransmitters as waste products (e.g., γ-aminobutyric acid [GABA]);

3. The production of short chain fatty acids [SCFA];

4. The production of useful metabolites such as niacin which reduces inflammation of the intestinal tract;

5. The use of the amino acid catabolism of tryptophan leads to bioactive molecules, which are endogenous ligands of several receptors regulating immune and inflammatory responses;

6. The production of a series of antimicrobial molecules (antibiotics of various origins, etc.) that aid competition among different species.

But the holobiont is formed out of microbes consisting also of viruses. Some viruses, called bacteriophages (or phages), live inside their bacterial hosts. So, these phages are bacterial viruses and do not attack human cells. Phages are obligate parasites of bacteria and bacteria have many mechanisms of defense against bacteriophage infection. Phages are the most abundant biological entities on Earth, with 70% of bacteria being infected. This huge number of phage particles also confirm the relative abundance of viruses in the human body (see Figure 2).

Phages can also transmit information from one bug to the other. This is the mechanism for antibiotic resistance, for example. This occurs since bacteriophages engage in the horizontal gene transfer, although there are other methods used by the microbiota to transmit information interspecies. We shall not discuss these as too technical.

Figure 2. Composition of the Human Holobiont (Percentage)

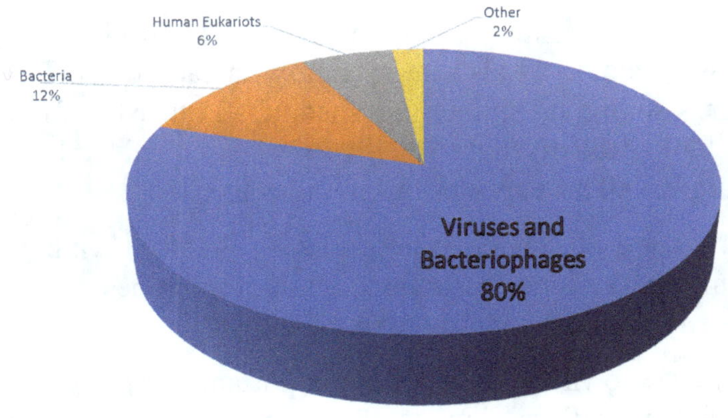

3.3.2 The Equilibrium

Now, if we wanted to take into consideration the global accumulated genetic makeup of the holobiont (the host [human being] and relative resident microbes), we would understand what's going on inside a human being.

Non-human genes, i.e., those belonging to the microbes, can synthetize enzymes that are helpful for a set of activities which cannot be done by us as humans, like breaking down some specific fibers.

Non-human genes can be brought (or introduced voluntarily) into human cells, via different mechanisms. Now the consequences of this may seem to be long lasting.

The holobiont is a metaorganism (the concentration of multiple organisms living in symbiosis [happily helping each other] with one another).

As a consequence of this view, viruses then should not be considered as always pathogenic for everyone in every case. No, that is an incorrect way of thinking, since in the light of the holobiont, they share their fate with that of their hosts. Viruses, like all other microorganisms establish complex interaction networks within their living ecosystem (our own tissues).

The holobiont is inherently composed of multiple species living "together" as a whole and also interacting with each other. Their vast number is so high to simply overshadow all other life forms. Also, their biological diversity (biodiversity) is equally great as viruses can infect all host species (all living cells).

Viruses have now been fully recognized as also symbiotic (assisting) members of the host's association of microbes. Viruses adapt to the environment and can do many things.

There are a few known functions of the importance of gut viruses within the gut microflora. Among the functions are also those involved in using and storing energy, such as for carbohydrate transport and degradation (destruction into little usable food compounds). Yet other benefits of viruses are the supply of immunity to infection by bacterial pathogens (bad bugs), and commensal bacteria (good bugs). This in turn stimulates beneficial functions like immunity.

Let's not forget that there is a link between the brain (host part) and the gut function (microbiota): the famous brain-gut axis. Some significant functions include the neuro-immune system, and the production of neurological metabolites (waste products), such as serotonin, noradrenalin.

The holobiont then results from the staggeringly high and precise symbiotic interactions between the microbial associates, including viruses, and a host, which can impact important host traits.

3.3.3 Conclusions

An amazing new world has been discovered and surely enough this will impact our view of health habits, forever. From the analysis of all the data concerning the metaorganism/holobiont as a gathering of dependent organisms, a clear though complex picture of the existence of the holobiont has been drawn. Nothing within us is sterile. On the contrary, everything we know confirms that we are in homeostasis or symbiosis (helping relationship) with our own microorganisms.

The following conclusions can be described:

1. There is an enormous amount of biochemical and biophysical interactions with feedback loops between host and microbiota;

2. The perfect alignment between every niche-resident microbiota and host-relative tissue confirms that we are highly designed creatures;

3. All microorganisms living within a single human body are original and unique to its host biochemical make-up (physical structure);

4. Any variation, whether natural or not, will affect the established equilibrium;

5. All forms of host diseases are seen as a dysbiosis of some sort (disequilibrium with the bugs) which interferes with

the normal interactions between the host and its resident microbiota (normal living bugs).

More conclusions can be illustrated, obviously, but this is to show how important bugs are truly to us all.

3.4 Small Carbohydrates (Glycans)

Carbohydrates are essentially sugars. Short- or long-chained, it makes little difference if they can be destroyed by our own enzymes into their base components. Carbohydrates are the most complex of all macromolecules (big molecules: proteins, DNA, etc.). We need though to be reminded that what small carbohydrates are, should not be called sugars or carbohydrates. The important difference with sugars and carbohydrates is that these special molecules are more like fibers (undigestible or cannot be destroyed by our own enzymes). They are also sometimes called glycans, especially the short-chained ones. Why are they so special? Well, because of:

1. Their complexity with properties such as:

    a. Their variety;

    b. Their different "bond type";

    c. Their different "bond position" (3D structure).

Each of these properties grants the carbohydrate a unique type of complexity that makes them far superior to all other macromolecules. While proteins and nucleic acids (DNA and RNA) are linear in their structure, glycans are not. This is a result of the "bond position". Now, let's look at the complexity of these small carbohydrates.

3.4.1 Variety of Glycans

The pieces of a sequence of carbohydrates, normally called glycans (like Lego pieces, but chemically called sugar monomers or monosaccharides), come in many different shapes and forms. This distinction depends on the wild variety of their chemical structure. Indeed, there are so many of these base constituents that the alphabet (with 22 letters) was insufficient to clearly distinguish each one of them. Hence, it was hence necessary to develop a new system of identification to represent them graphically. This system had to be both easy and intuitive to quickly visualize and understand each base constituent. A cartoon illustration was created with colored boxes, and triangles and other simple geometric figures. Each of these figures represented a specific base carbohydrate (hereafter called just "monomers", from the fact that they are single [mono] compounds). This system is used to represent these base constituents or monomers and is called "Cartoon Representation of Glycans". Most of them are shown schematically in Table 1, with their respective colors.

Table 1. Table of Reference for Carbohydrate Monomers

SHAPE	White (Generic)	Blue	Green	Yellow	Orange	Pink	Purple	Light Blue	Brown	Red
Filled Circle	Hexose	Glc	Man	Gal	Gul	Alt	All	Tal	Ido	
Filled Square	HexNAc	GlcNAc	ManNAc	GalNAc	GulNAc	AltNAc	AllNAc	TalNAc	IdoNAc	
Crossed Square	Hexosamine	GlcN	ManN	GalN	GulN	AltN	AllN	TalN	IdoN	
Divided Diamond	Hexuronate	GlcA	ManA	GalA	GulA	AltA	AllA	TalA	IdoA	
Filled Triangle	Deoxyhexose	Qui	Rha		6dGul	6dAlt		6dTal		Fuc
Divided Triangle	DeoxyhexNAc	QuiNAc	RhaNAc			6dAltNAc		6dTalNAc		FucNAc
Flat Rectangle	Di-deoxyhexose	Oli	Tyv		Abe	Par	Dig	Col		
Filled Star	Pentose		Ara	Lyx	Xyl	Rib				
Filled Diamond	Deoxynonulosonate		Kdn				Neu5Ac	Neu5Gc	Neu	Sia
Flat Diamond	Di-deoxynonulosonate		Pse	Leg		Aci		4eLeg		
Flat Hexagon	Unknown	Bac	LDmanHep	Kdo	Dha	DDmanHep	MurNAc	MurNGc	Mur	
Pentagon	Assigned	Api	Fru	Tag	Sor	Psi				

I say most of them because the actual number is larger, although the others are quite rare. Nevertheless, the ones here presented amount to a total of 70! an impressive number, if you think that these are carbohydrates and outnumber almost 4 times that of proteins.

Just looking at the number of glycans we can already say that the linear sequence of carbohydrates can be almost 4 times more complex that proteins. But this is not the most intricate part of them! No, this is the least fascinating and complex-adding facet. The best part is the branching of the sequence (not linear anymore but cleft)! This branching of glycan superstructures is not limited to just 1 position for each monomer but up to 5 positions can be used. This means that branching does not just confer a doubling of the complexity but up to 4/5 times more with respect to the same number of pieces of amino acids (proteins) or nucleotides (DNA/RNA).

Allow me to clarify this with a simple example. Let's take a protein and a fragment of DNA composed by a sequence of 5 identical monomers (aa or nucleotides) as is the case. Because of their linear order there will be only 1 possible form (say, AAAAA): no permutations or other multiplicity is allowed. A hypothetical 5 monomer glycan (pentasaccharide), on the other hand, will have multiple forms, each of which is different from the other and cannot be compared to or identified with the others. They would be distinct, diverse entities, period. Check out Figure 3.

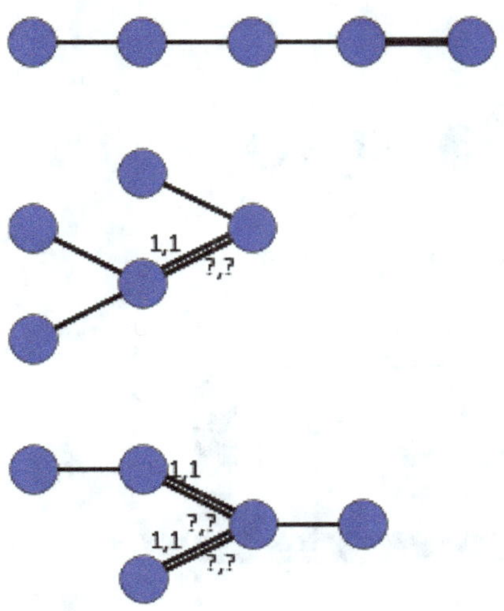

As can be easily seen, apart from the first sequence, which is linear and mimics proteins and DNA/RNA, the others are more complex. The first linear structure is normally called "BASIC" with normal α1-4 bonds (the simplest glycan bond type). But α1-4 bonds do not need to be necessarily present. Other bond types do exist, such as α1-2, or α1-3, α1-5 up to α1-6 (in certain cases) and can be "used". You see how complex these do become. Add to this that there are two types of glycosidic bonds, and we have a super complex molecule. These other bonds are 1,4 alpha and 1,4 beta glycosidic bonds. I won't explain their spatial nature. So just trust me, they are specular but different.

Without bothering you any further on showing other essential sugars and their possible structures, I will just help you notice that there is practically no limit in the variability of the structure of glycans as presented in Figure 4.

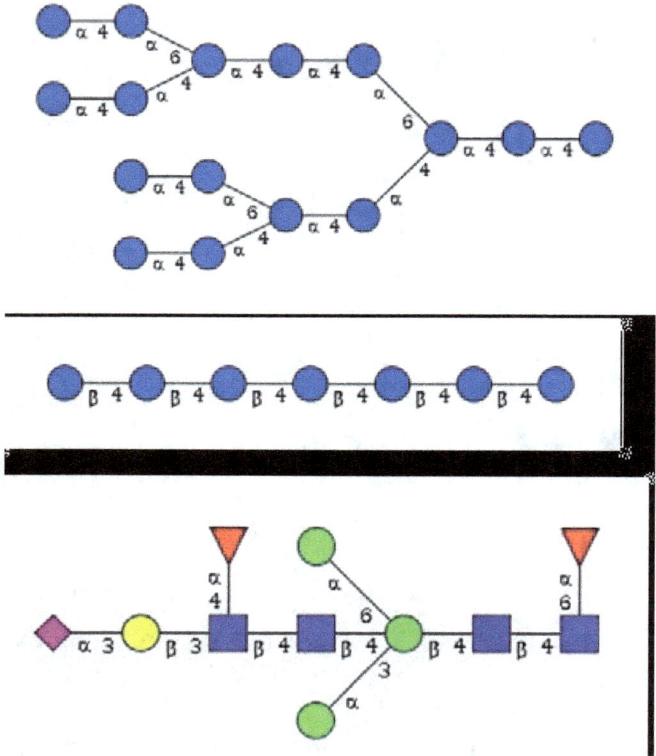

In this figure, there are three carbohydrates, of which two fibers. The first structure represents a branched starch (glucose) with its α1-4 and 1-6 glycosidic linkages. The second is the structure of a cellulose (glucose) with its β1-4 glycosidic bond (fiber). The third is a cartoon representation of a simple (linear) glycan with many linkage types between several different saccharide residues.

p. 34/193

3.4.2 Ubiquitousness (they are everywhere)

It is hard to break it to most people how small yet powerful are these biochemical compounds. As they normally say, when people tell them that ABO type diets are effective, that: "No, it's not true. It only acts on the blood, not on the whole body" or other similar reactions. But this is a very false conception of the biochemistry of glycans! Indeed, ABO determinants are glycans. And it is worst when such startling declarations come from physicians or other self-called scientists. The reality is merely much more complex.

In fact, we need to realize that glycans are everywhere in biological systems (nature). All cells, yes you are reading this correctly, all cells have a structure on top of their membrane which is called glycocalyx constituted of glycans linked to other biological structures (proteins or lipids).

Figure 5. Schematic Representation of a Cell Membrane

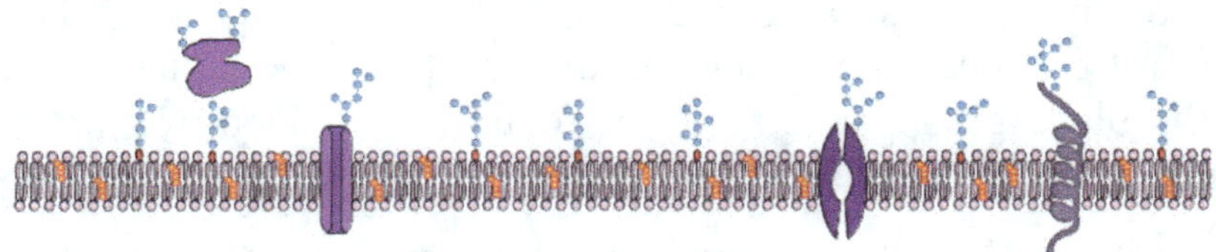

The blue marbles that are on top of the purple proteins and the pinkish membrane, are glycans.

Glycans in blue circles (or marbles) are bound to other structures like proteins (purple) or phospholipids (pinkish) present on the cell membrane. Thus, all cells are literally coated with these peculiar carbohydrates.

3.4.3 ABO Blood Groups

The ABO blood group determinants (another name for antigens or epitopes [biochemical compounds that react with certain molecules]) are glycans. ABO glycans have a specific change at the ending epitope (a glycan A or a glycan B), that differentiates them structurally, chemically, and biochemically.

p. 35/193

These antigens were first discovered in the blood giving the proper name to this system of classifying these determinants. It was the Austrian pathologist Karl Landsteiner in 1901, who discovered and classified the blood groups based on the presence of A and B antigens on the surface of red blood cells. This is the reason why they are called "blood" groups (due to them being found on the red blood cells).

The classical view of the ABO antigens is that of modulation of how our body responds to stimuli in the blood. Indeed, during the first transfusions, it was noticed that different people having different types of bloods display diverse immune properties. What happened was that antibodies in the plasma of one blood group reacted with antigens on the surfaces of the red blood cells of another blood type (or vice versa).

This fact which was being studied and demonstrated repeatedly led to the hypothesis that the ABO blood determinants are features of the red blood cells alone. But this concept was only much later discarded as deemed unfounded. And this delay led to the idea that ABO blood groups could only be found in the blood. Nothing is further from the truth!

Since the ABO blood group is the most important blood group system (being linked to transfusions and transplantation), it is also thought to be the only one. Notwithstanding this, the ABO blood groups have a central role because of its unique biochemical characteristics, which will be described hereafter.

Do not worry, it will be easy to understand as I will use the aid of pictures to simplify the comprehension of the essential features of this special glycans.

There are four basic ABO phenotypes (scientific word for constitution) that derive from the three ABO determinants (see Figure 6). The four phenotypes correspond to the four ABO blood grouping: these are O, A, B, and AB.
As we mentioned earlier, the ABO blood groups are defined by carbohydrate moieties (another word for molecular structure)

which are displayed on the surface of red blood cells and attached to a protein or a lipid backbone. These macro (big) molecules (because composed of more than one molecule [glycan and protein or lipid]) are known as "glycoconjugates". The O antigen (also called as the H antigen in several texts [so don't worry if you see around ABH, it means ABO – we won't use it here if only sparingly]) is the basis on which the other two groups are formed by additional glycosylation. These are genetically determined.

As you can see for yourself in Figure 6, the O antigen (number 3) is the smallest glycan of the three ABO determinants.

Figure 6. ABO Determinants (Glyco-chemistry)

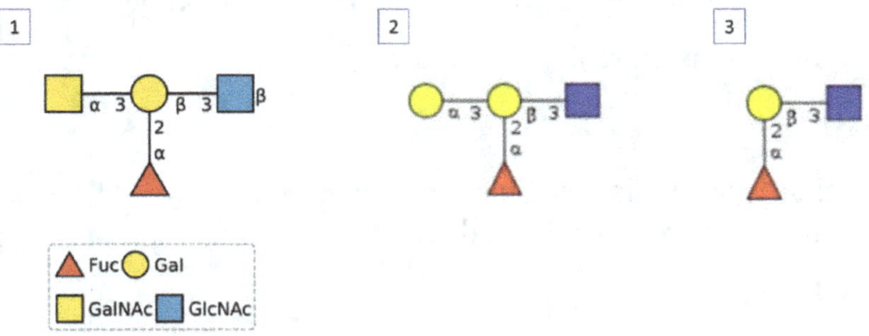

As shown previously, the color-coded geometric figures represent a peculiar monosaccharide (sugar derivative), and the three-letter name of the glycan or sugar monomer is presented next to the figure. 1 is A, 2 is B and 3 is O.

These glycans, being everywhere in the human body, do have long-ranging effects both biochemically and biologically. We shall see this in the next section.

3.4.4 The ABO -Food Interaction

We have seen how different these ABO glycans are and where they are in the human body (on top of all cells and where proteins and fats are present). Now we shall see what they can do.

Because they are molecules, they can react with other molecules surrounding them. Certain proteins, called lectins, can recognize, and bind only to specific glycans based on their physical and chemical structure (3D spatial disposition of atoms). Even microbes do prefer (because of their enzymatic background) some glycans and not others.

Given these facts (all scientifically proven), it is evident that food is perfectly capable of interacting at a molecular level with our biomolecules, according to a specific pattern. Food thus reacts with glycans, either soluble in body fluids or bound to the cell membrane and may bring about an immune or inflammatory response or not. Based on this, there is a perfectly scientific reason as to why the body handles certain foods, stress, and illnesses differently than someone with a different ABO blood type.

Actually, there is more than one reason.

3.4.4.1 *Mechanism One*

The first reason is the classical mechanism of ABO-food interaction: the presence of food lectins.

These food lectins:

1. are present in the diet and resist heat and digestion;
2. are capable of recognizing and binding to different glycans with different strengths;
3. show polyvalent behaviour (depend on the concentration of glycans);
4. may not bind to masked glycans, i.e., spatially impeded by similar sugar residues such as blood group determinants or sialic acids.

But this is only one part of the whole picture. Amazingly science has discovered recently other reasons as we shall now see. There are two new mechanisms by which food can interfere with the normal homeostatic processes and induce a stress.

3.4.4.2 *Mechanism Two*

The second reason is that glycans are also present in food stuff. And this is something that should be obvious to everyone but has never been previously brought up as a scientific argument. It has been confirmed by several experiments that glycans not only are present in foods but are also used by microorganisms in the gut. So, they do pass intact the acidic environment of the stomach. Once in the gut, food glycans can either:

- interact with the human lectins. Proteins are present in humans and can bind to glycans. Examples of these lectins are galectin-4 or -8, immune proteins present in the GI tract, or

- interact with glycans of various types on the cell membranes in the gut. The major cells are enterocytes, or

- be absorbed into the internal milieu and presented to the immune system cells where they can react and

thus, elicit an immune or inflammatory response, not only in the first bullet point, but in all three cases.

There is no need to go into many details of the immune system structure of the gut and of the human body. What is true is that this is something that has been shown extensively to occur in scientific experiments. Now, what is the difference between diverse ABO blood types?

Simple, because blood glycans are present everywhere they can react differently with these chemical compounds. Glycans can:

1. interact with human lectins, as ABO specific glycan-binding proteins on the top of cells. The affinity, specificity and strength of these interactions can be defined by:

   a) the presence of ABO specific clustered saccharide patch, where several closely spaced glycans interact to generate a specific recognition epitope. A spatial formation of proteins and fats that is unique depending on the ABO glycans;

b) the presence of lipid rafts, in the form of specific cell surface domains, where proteins and glycans may be clustered (grouped) together to allow for multiple interactions;

2. interact with human ABO or other glycans on the cell membrane of enterocytes;

3. interact with soluble ABO specific lectins or immunoglobulins with the same modalities as outlined earlier.

Once such interaction is established, the formation of special cross-linking between lectins, such as galectins, and proteins, called lattices, may be favoured, or impeded depending on the particular functional and spatial conformation of the membrane lipid rafts formed.

The lipid rafts, I mentioned earlier are formed by the presence of glycans that interact with other glycans present on fats (glycolipids) and on proteins (glycoproteins). As shown in Figure 7, the ABO specific glycans (blue dots) drive the "closing in" (the grouping, the assembly) only of certain macromolecules (glycoproteins and glycolipids).

The lipid raft allows proteins on the cell membrane to be assembled with a preferred conformation where they were previously far across. This occurs essentially because the glycans can form special protein to carbohydrate or carbohydrate to carbohydrate interactions with specific proteins, spatially close to them.

Figure 7. Formation of a Lipid Raft

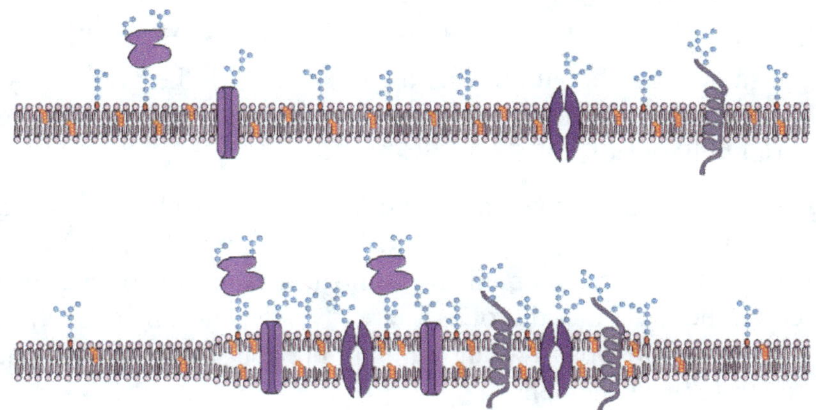

The figure identifies two cell membrane where the phospholipids act as the base layer and the glycans (small bluish dots) are linked to either the phospholipids or the glycoproteins (purple transmembrane structures).

Glycolipids and glycoproteins thereafter come together to co-operate differentially with other glycoproteins or glycolipids based on the ABO glycans present. It is only at this point that the formation of these lipid raft can initiate a signal transduction. A signal that is sent molecularly with the cell. These signal pathways can produce several effects, among which are those for immune cell activation.

3.4.4.3 *Mechanism Three*

The third mechanism is the influence of food item glycans on the microbiota. Since the gut contains approximately 10–100 trillion microorganisms, which include 100–200 different bacterial species, this must affect the host's health condition.

Specifically, plant and animal glycans, can be selectively foraged (eaten) by the certain microorganisms. As a result, there will be an alteration of the microbial composition in the intestinal lumen, because those that can eat the glycans will survive. And this alteration will affect the metabolic activities of the microbes. Hence, certain microbes will be favoured with respect to others

p. 41/193

based on their enzymatic toolbox in degrading and obtaining energy from glycans. Of course, this ability (enzymatic activity) allows them to grow faster than the others and survive or thrive.

In the same way, the gut, has its own glycans (on the glycocalyx, cell membrane), to offer to the microbes as readily available material to harvest for their survival.

Again, only those species of microbes with the right enzymatic toolbox will thrive while the other will die. Since ABO groups are glycans, different microorganisms will survive (or just be present) based on the ABO blood groups. Here, the ABO group connection with the microflora has a wealth of literature and scientific data that corroborate this statement.

Now, it becomes logical to deduce that when the right species of microorganisms survive due to the right diet (ABO similar glycans) and ABO group, our gut is healthy. On the contrary, when microbes are present due to the wrong diet and they do not agree with our ABO group, our health deteriorates causing many a disease.

It is a well-known fact that the food in our diet has an effect on the composition of species of the microbiota. Less known, though equally scientifically proven, is the fact that both are reciprocally influenced by the ABO group characteristic of the host.

To my knowledge, this third mechanism, while already known and considered mainstream science for some years, has never been used as a proof of concept of nor applied to the ABO diet (food-ABO link).

Both mechanisms can invoke a new discovery made in glycoscience in recent years. The existence of carbohydrate-to-carbohydrate interaction (CCI). That is, a novel mechanism proposed explain how spatially near proteins can further interact with each other.

This mechanism is schematically shown in Figure 8.

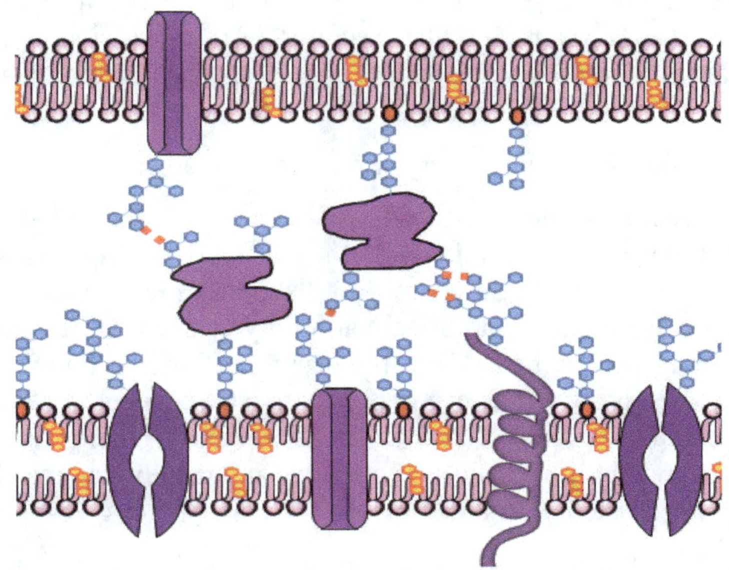

Red arrows indicate where the CCI (red dotted lines) from two different glycan molecules establish an almost covalent binding pattern. The strength is obviously inferior to that of a covalent bond but still strong enough to affect the shape of a protein or the interaction between two proteins on two different cell membranes.

Figure 8 explains graphically how two cell membranes, one belonging to the human body (e.g., a gut cell) and the other a microorganism (e.g., a bug), can interact in a highly specific and differential way. All depending on the host's blood type.

Thus, food items can pharmacologically interact with specific receptors and manifest as biologically active substances, which may regulate or dis-regulate physiologic processes in ways well beyond our current understanding.

3.4.5 The Final ABO-Food Scheme

One last thing that we should consider is the variability of the ABO blood typing within the human body.

3.4.5.1 _Variabilities_

There are other glycans similar to ABO but clearly different: the Lewis (Le) glycans and the Secretor (Se) expression of these glycans. I shall not go into details of these as they have been amply explained by several authors in the past few years.

ABO and Le glycans are very similar to each other.

This identifies the first level of variability since the ABO phenotype imposes limitations to the type of glycans being expressed by Le and Se genes. But also, both Lewis and Secretor type impose the first additional variability on the manifestation of such glycans in humans. To better clarify, both Lewis and Secretor type can be positive (**Le** or **Se**) or negative (**le** or **se**, not expressing a particular glycan). This difference clearly manifests itself phenotypically (physically-structurally) and then biochemically in any related reaction (interaction with proteins, other glycans, etc.).

An example of the ABO and Lewis positive ABH antigens are shown in Figure 9.

Figure 9. Similitude between ABH Blood and Lewis antigens

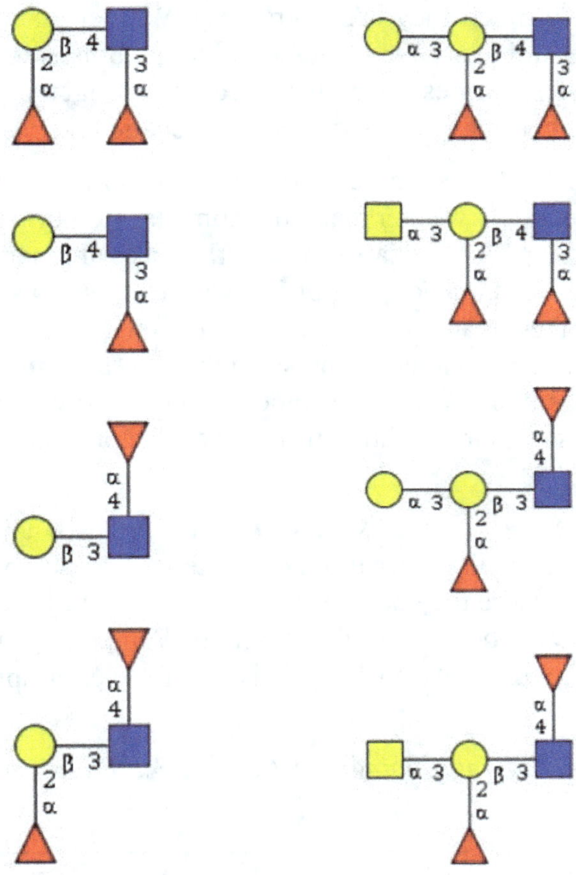

The antigens shown in this Figure are Lewis determinants (from left to right). The first two lines are Type 2 chains, while the last two lines are Type 1 chains. Starting from the bottom up you can see: on the first line from the bottom, on the left Lewis B (similar to the blood group H [or O] antigen with the additional fucosyl group on the GlcNAc residue), and A Lewis A (similar to the blood group A antigen with the additional fucosyl group on the GlcNAc residue); on the second line first line Lewis A determinant (precursor of Lewis B antigen) and B Lewis B (similar to B antigen but with an additional fucosyl group on the GlcNAc residue); the third line from the bottom represents a Lewis X (precursor of Lewis Y having a fucosyl group on the GlcNAc residue at the α1-3 position) and a A Lewis Y (similar to A antigen with a fucosyl group on the GlcNAc residue at the α1-3 position); finally, the first line from the top includes Lewis Y (structurally similar to H [or O] antigen but with the GlcNAc fucosylated in α1-3) and a B Lewis Y (similar to the B determinant).

p. 45/193

This first level of additional variability is then further surpassed by another level of variability identified by the variants of the A and B antigens (how much they are expressed). Weaker phenotypes of both A and B antigens have been identified in humans where these glycans are less expressed with respect to stronger phenotypes. These phenotypes have been studied at a genetic level.

Experiments conducted on humans have shown that all rare A and B subgroups display weaker reactivity compared to normal (strong) A or B blood type individuals. These differences are manifested as a distribution or frequency of A or B glycan expression so much as to give weaker reactions or to be nonreactive serologically. Moreover, these individuals expressing these weaker subgroups of A or B can easily be mistyped as blood group O individuals. Blood O individuals miss the additional sugar residue present in A and B blood types.

Indeed, those people with weaker genetic A or B antigen will phenotypically display ever more characteristics resembling an O blood type the more they have distant numberings or letters to A or B and thus will be closer to a combined/ mixed constitution: something like an A/O and B/O. This can be seen graphically in Figure 10.

Figure 10. ABO Subgrouping Spectrum (A and B antigens)

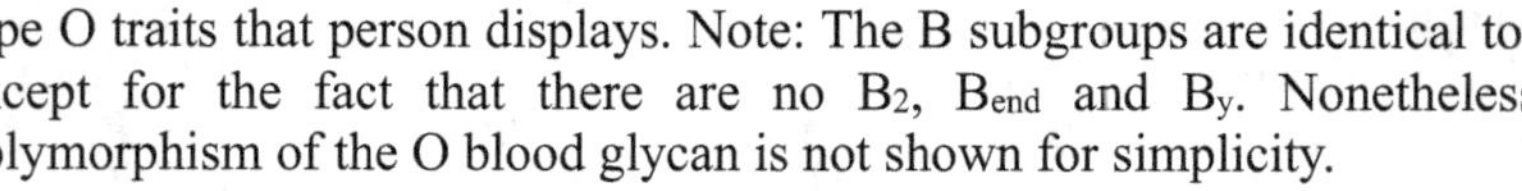

$$A_1 \qquad A_2, A_3, A_x, A_{end}, A_m, A_y, A_{el}, \quad O \quad B_{el}, \quad B_m, \quad B_x, \qquad B_3 \quad B$$

The Figure clearly classifies people having subgroupings with higher numbers or letters on a spectrum of distribution. On this spectrum, the centre is the O blood type and the closer to this a person with a subgrouping is the more blood type O traits that person displays. Note: The B subgroups are identical to the A except for the fact that there are no B_2, B_{end} and B_y. Nonetheless, the polymorphism of the O blood glycan is not shown for simplicity.

To visualize this graphically, weaker phenotypes on a continuum and their 'relative' closeness to (distance from) the O blood group (in descending order of site density from the point of the arrows).

It has been argued that the closer the subgrouping to O a person has, the more the person displays phenotypically the biochemical and physiologic traits of a blood type O. This results directly from the CCI and PCI on the glycocalyx of the cells in the human body, whether in the blood or not.

Within the ABO subgroups, the weaker phenotypes of both A and B antigens are experimentally demonstrated on the erythrocytes to easily be mistyped as blood group O individuals: they do give weaker reactions or are nonreactive serologically with anti B antisera.

This overall variability (or heterogeneity) is a peculiar attribute of this typology, and it also allows for the easy identification of a biological marker to assess the influence of genetic factors of the individual. Personalized medicine can thus become much easier in the future once these techniques are utilized ever so abundantly by nutritionists and physicians.

3.4.5.2 *The Scheme*

These newly proposed mechanisms have now to be included into a final explanatory scheme.

The last figure (Figure 11) represents the summary of all afore mentioned scientifically proven statements, as presented in literature across several fields of science. The figure does clarify how much and how complex these interactions provoke reactions within the human body.

Foods per se contain substances (lectins and glycans) that will influence (interact and reversibly bind) both microbial and gut cell surface glycans and proteins (receptors). Once bound they can thereby trigger appropriate biological responses.

Figure 11. Proven relationship between ABO blood group and Food

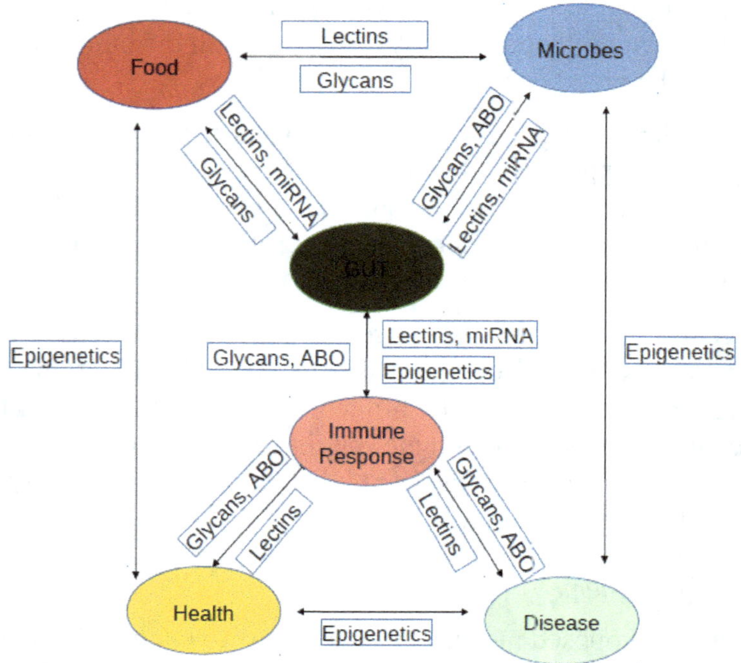

When lectins are displayed it is to be intended proteins and glycans together.

Whether the food, it has been shown that these molecules can affect their biochemical action selectively in the presence of certain ABO glycans. Again, the microbiota (belly bugs) is closely linked and selected by the ABO group of the host, so that it is possibly to state and affirm the following relationship:

Food influences the micobiota → microbiota is tailored by and for the host's ABO group → the ABO antigens decide which foods are good.

The particular chemical structure of foods can activate signal transduction pathways in gut cells or proteins and thus generate a series of biological responses. And it all depends on the genetic and epigenetic make-up of the individual (ABO, etc.).

p. 48/193

From all the vast literature available, the following statements can be used to summarize the status:

1. if a food is recognized as bad it will elicit an immune or inflammatory response,

2. alternatively, if a food is accepted as good or neutral, little or no such event will be evoked;

3. the immune or inflammatory reaction is mediated by cells within the ABO blood group system;

4. microorganisms present in the gut may impact on health/ disease through the ABO antigen system;

5. Genetic diversity (ABO) rules, so that everybody is unique;

6. Genetic diversity (ABO) determines which foods are allowed (good/ neutral) and which are not (bad).

It has been noted that certain food items are harmful regardless of the blood group of an individual. Among these, it was possible to characterize them in different classes as follows:

1. Always harmful: cereals (especially gluten-containing) and milk (non-human milk);

2. harmful when taken in higher quantities and/ or frequencies: fruits and sugary substances (honey, etc.);

3. Harmful and beneficial depending on the ABO type;

4. Always beneficial, if not consumed in large quantities and if no allergy is present: salmon, egg, water.

And finally, of course, there is the individual genetic variance in everyone that makes us unique. This calls for personalized diet and nutritional plans to consider the various intolerances and variabilities of each individual.

p. 49/193

3.5 Ancient Biotypes

The definition of individual constitution (biotype) was a very ancient question, as the various medical theories have tackled this from the beginning. The nature of human temperament was already formed in the Ionic philosophy at the time of Hippocrates. Over the years, his medical activity, developed from several keen observations, was systematized in a version that remained a reference paradigm during many centuries.

The term constitution (physique or body-build or somatotype) refers to the total sum of an individual's morphological, physiological, psychological, and immunological attributes. These may be determined mainly by hereditary influences of some form or another (genetic and epigenetic [close to genes but not quite]). Hence, disease results from the interplay of various external factors to which our organism reacts. Each patient has a constellation of disease-causing factors differing in grouping from that of every other patient.

We will now define the historical context in which temperament and constitution did evolve in the following sections.

3.5.1 The origin

The notion of "temperament" can be traced back to the ancient times. The traditions of ancient Egypt and Mesopotamia (1500 BC) recount that the health of the human body was co connected with the four basic elements of nature—fire, water, soil, and air. This can also be traced back into the Book of Ezekiel in the Bible.

3.5.1.1 <u>Ancient Times</u>

The origin of the four-fold division of elements could be based on Empedocles's (495-430 BC) theories or Heraclitus (540-475 BC), and Alcmaeon of Crotona (510 BC). Most of these physicians believed that disease was the result of the imbalance of essential opposites, hot and cold, dry, and wet, etc.

Hippocrates is considered the founder of constitutional investigation and studies of interrelationship between morphology and susceptibility to disease. Hippocrates offered two-fold classification of physique (somatotyping). "Habitus phthisicus", long and thin individuals, the first and "Habitus apoplecticus", short and thick build individuals, the second.

According to Hippocrates, the physician had to examine a patient, observe symptoms carefully, make a diagnosis and then treat the patient. It is incredible to notice how advanced was the Hippocratic medical science. The concept of stressors founded in the work of Walter Cannon and Hans Selye, the maintenance of homeostasis, the rediscovery of the importance of food and the body-mind link are but a few of its achievements.

Even the simple concept that food is an alternative to medicine, typical of Hippocratic practitioners, has had a long and difficult road towards acceptance. Indeed, Hippocrates' famous "Let food be thy medicine and medicine be thy food" philosophy can be used at least in preventive medicine.

Aristotle (384-322 BC) in his book "Physiognomica" tried to find a correlation between the external lineaments of man and his mental and moral characteristics. Aristotle is held as the writer of the lengthy treatise on the art of reading traits from faces.

The Graeco-Roman medicine was permeated by the notion that disease results from an imbalance of the four humours. This concept persisted until the eighteenth century, when it was superseded by more 'scientific' doctrines (sic).

This theory of humors and temperaments spread well beyond western civilization in space and time. It became incorporated in other traditional medicines.

It was not until the Roman physician, surgeon, and philosopher Galen of Pergamon (130 AD-210 AD) that these notions were codified. Galen being a master at rhetoric with impeccable logic, was also a prolific writer and spread the humoral theory throughout much of the known world.

3.5.1.2 *Middle Ages and Beyond*

During the middle ages, it was widely used in both Europe and in the Middle East.

In Europe, the first European medical school was opened in Salerno, Italy and a slightly altered four humors theory emerged. The Salerno Medical School upheld not only the main principle of humoral theory of Hippocrates and Galen, but also the writings of Constantine the African homeopathy.

Avicenna (Ibn Sina also known as, c. 980 AD-1037 AD, the well-known Persian physician and philosopher) wrote "The Qanon of Medicine". It was based on Iranian traditional medicine system with its balancing of the humors in the human body. Avicenna was also a pioneer of clinical trials, antedating modern clinical trials by one millennium. The Canon of Medicine was a true medical encyclopedia and brought him fame for centuries.

In the middle ages, the medical knowledge was pass down through Europe and the Middle East. Some notable figures are reported with reference to their involvement in the spreading of these concepts.

William Shakespeare (1564-1616), perhaps the most important and influent writer of English tradition, frequently referenced and wrote characters with specific humoral temperaments. Examples of such humoral characteristic are Hamlet (melancholy), Sir John Falstaff (phlegmatic), Lady Macbeth (choleric), and Viola (sanguine).

In the late eighteenth and early nineteenth century in France, Halle and Rostan described three types of physical constitutions as "digestif", "musculaire" and "cerebrale". The French School of Biotypology had its early founder in Noel Halle (1754-1822).

p. 52/193

Similarly, several writers and thinkers have used ancient concepts (like the four temperaments) and expanded on them as they seemed fit.

Kant, the greatest philosopher of modern times, developed a system of ethics based on the four humours of ancient derivation. Kant derived his knowledge from thinkers like Hugo de Folieto (Hugh of Fouilloy, 1111-1172), Jean Baptist Moliere (playwriter, 1622-1673), Christian Thomasius (jurist, 1655-1728), moralists like Jean de Le Bruyère (1645-1696), doctors like Michael Medina (1564), when referring directly to poet and physiognomist Jean Casper Lavater (1741-1801), anthropologist and physician Ernst Platner (1744-1818) and writer Adolph Freiherr Knigge (1752-1796).

3.5.1.3   *19th – 20th Century*

One of the last great teachers of Galen's doctrine was none other than Professor Thomas Laycock (1812-1876), English physician and neurophysiologist.

The concept of the four humors and temperaments survived even until the twentieth century when they found their way to modern psychology. In the 19th century, medicine was still dominated by the humoral doctrine. But the development of the germ theory of disease (bacteriology and medical parasitology) signed the emergence of medical modernity.

Neo-humoralism and neo-Hippocratism, was still very strong late into the twentieth century.

I shall not endeavor to describe all theories as they are simply too many. I shall just touch upon some more modern scientists, like the psychiatrist Ernst Kretschmer (1888 AD - 1964 AD) and William H. Sheldon (1898 AD - 1977) Sheldon classified humans into three categories according to their body shape. These categories are:

1. endomorphs (having a slow metabolism);

2. mesomorphs (with a normal metabolism), and

3.   ectomorphs (with accelerated metabolism).

Kretschmer in 1921 submitted his theory of the biological affinity between the psychic disposition and body build. His four constitutions were the pyknic (excessive breadth in relation to length), the athletic (strong development of muscular system), the leptosomatic (or asthenic, thin but long bones) and dysplastic physiques.

In more recent times, Paul Hindemith formulated his philosophy of music upon the concept of the four temperaments of historical importance. In October 1940 Hindemith composed an almost thirty-minute set of four tripartite variations on a tripartite theme, intended for performance at the New York City Ballet. The end-result was a system of pairing tonal centers and religiously symbolic ideas and images with an overall theme linked to the medieval four temperaments of Galenic origin.

Probably the most important and influential modern writer that dabbled with the four temperaments is the psychologist Carl Jung. Jungian character and personality archetypes taken from the medieval past are linked to the psychology of individuation which he developed into his main theory.

At the beginning of the 20th century, physiognomy enjoyed renewed popularity. Some companies as AT&T, used physiognomy as one of their main tools in assessing candidates.

We will now proceed to delineate the theory in our times.

3.5.1.4   *Rest Of the World Diffusion*

In America, humoral medicine has been recognized by anthropologists to be a largely simplified folk variant of classical Greek and Persian humoral pathology. Contemporary folk medical beliefs and practices descended from classical Greek Hippocratic humoral pathology.

Rural Dominican humoral theory is one of the many doctrines that developed around the idea of clod/hot humors (taken from Hippocratic medicine).

In Asia, Sasang constitutional medicine (SCM) was developed, as a unique traditional Korean therapeutic alternative form of medicine.

In Europe, constitutional medicine was born in and around the 1920s. It gained ground during the 1930s by adding new principles to the 'science of the [human] constitutions, temperaments, and characters'.

Unani (the Arabic name for Greek) medicine is normally taught in specially recognized Universities in Pakistan, South Africa, Iran, Kuwait, and UAE, apart from India and China. It is officially recognized by the Health Authorities of those countries and by the WHO.

The humoral theory has spread beyond Europe to include the Arab nations, Latin America and even some Southeast Asian countries (Philippines and Malaysia), although with their own peculiar twist, but substantially maintaining its general principle).

Figure 12 shows the diffusion of constitutional medicines (traditional medicines) practices in the world but cross-influences are not considered, although it would highly be recommended.

p. 55/193

Figure 12.   Diffusion of Western and Eastern Traditional Medicines

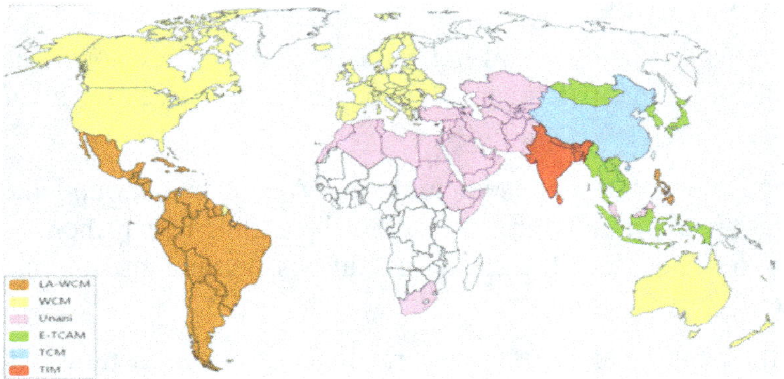

Robinson Projection Map for the diffusion of traditional medicines.

This map (Figure 12) shows the diffusion of various traditional medicines discussed around the World.

Beyond the 1940s, the neo-Hippocratic era faded away because official medicine was dominated by more interesting ideas.

3.5.2 Scientific Observations

Scientific approaches for physical constitution classification are based on the premise that physical constitutional features are expressed by face, body, voice, skin, pulse, and personality. Certain biotypes are endowed with slightly different biological processes, biochemical substrate variances and hormonal balances.

Many attempts have been made to validate the reasonableness of the humoral theory. Incredibly, most of these successful experiments come from scientists trying to demonstrate the effectiveness of Eastern Medicine.

3.5.2.1 *Human body composition*

The study of human body composition spans >100 y. It is continuing to be an active area of basic science and clinical research. The body shape, or somatotype (can be divided into the

p. 56/193

four components (bone mass, subcutaneous fat mass, muscle mass, and residual mass).

The study of human body composition is a branch of human biology which focuses on the in vivo quantification of body components. Various indices have been developed to meet the need of a more satisfactory objective method of distinguishing physical types.

Several modern studies have found links between the somatotype (mesomorphic, ectomorphic or endomorphic according to Sheldon and Heath-Carter) and diseases.

Constitution or biotype identifies a special mode of functioning of the endocrines and vegetative nervous system. It is modulated by the integrative system of the body, the pseudo-neuro-endocrine system.

Several clinical trials have been completed in the East to address the consistency of constitutional medicine as developed by TCM or Sasang biotypology.

A systematic review (and meta-analysis) of 11 clinical studies involving 12890 individuals was completed to find a correlation between Traditional Chinese Medicine (TCM) constitution and dyslipidemia. A meta-analysis is the highest level of clinical scientific evidence. The results demonstrated a significant predisposition of certain constitutions for the disease reviewed.

The discovery of chemical individuality by A. Garrod is a milestone in modern pharmacogenomics. With this concept genetic and chemical factors confer upon us the predisposition and immunities from diseases. This is confirmed by all observational data from recent clinical trials. We are now able to describe distinct profiles of individual patients and thus bring individualized care to patients.

3.5.2.2 *Humoral System*

The humoral system has seen many variants through time. There have been important differences in history between the initial

(Galen's) association of character traits and humours and the scheme of types that would become canonical in the centuries. In the early Middle Ages, there has not yet been a consistent characterization of phlegmatics and melancholics.

In the Commonwealth of Dominica, it is common knowledge that illness is the result of hot or cold humors that enter a person's body and disrupt the balance of his or her mental or physical state. This could occur through the environment by food (disruptive hot or cold forces) or injury, or by this form of medicine (bush medicine of hot/cold, humoral qualities).

According to this central American theory, five activities place the body in highly vulnerable situation:

- eating;

- bathing;

- menstruation: a time of above normal heat for women;

- exercise: after the heat a gradual cooling is recommended;

- sleeping: one has to cover up to avoid cold.

Maybe the most remarkable is the Unani system of medicine. Unani Tibb is the Arab version of the ancient western medicine. This was directly derived from Hippocratic and Galen's doctrines, with the addition of Avicenna's synthesis. The further development of Unani stressed the importance of prevention of disease and promotion of health rather than cure. There are six factors essential for the maintenance of good health:

1. Fresh Air;

2. Food and Drink;

3. Exercise and rest;

4. Mental health: psychological factors;

5. Sleep rhythm: good sleep;

6. Retention and Evacuation: regularity in the bathroom.

p. 58/193

3.5.2.3 _Similarities with other medical systems_

Apart from the already cited examples, the humoral theory of medicine can be found in various forms in other medicines.

Notable is the example of Tibetan medicines. Sowa Rigpa (gso ba rig pa), which means the 'Science of Healing', is the term used in the vernacular in all regions where Tibetan medicine has merged with local knowledge. In Tibetan medicine, as in most traditional medicines, the five basic elements, earth, water, fire, air (wind), and space, make up the three principal energies of life, or the three humors:

a) rlung, "wind" or "mobile energy";

b) mkrispa, "bile", is composed of fire; and

c) badken phlegm, is composed of the elements of earth and water.

Here again, the four basic constitutions are summed up and become evident from the three Tibetan humors, with one being composed of two basic elements.

Although not essentially the same, constitutional types of therapeutic systems have also been devised.

An illustrious example is Iridology. A British iridology organization states that there are three main "constitutional types" of iris color:

- The blue-eyed constitution ("lymphatic type"),

- The "pure brown eyed constitution ("haematogenic type")

- The combination of the two ("mixed, dyscratic or biliary type")

Although alternative practitioners describe substantial success with the iris diagnosis, conventional medicine is not convinced. This may be due to the subjective interpretation of the diagnostic method (what is seen in the iris image).

p. 59/193

Similarly, traditional Chinese medicine (TCM) divided humans into:

- Balanced constitution, also known as Normality ("Pinghe" in Chinese) constitution, and

- Unbalanced/Biased ("Pianpo" in Chinese) constitution, which can be further classified into several other subtypes.

This is interesting because there may be an explanation confirming these differences. Indeed, different types of TCM constitutions may be seen as the aggravation of specific characteristics of the unbalanced type. Each subtype has their own peculiar physical, physiological, psychological, and pathological reaction states, it is likely that the constitution of a subtype is the dominated by on characteristic (e.g., metabolism).

Here again we may look into the category of four biotypes and dismiss the other 4/5 somatotypes (subtypes), due to their status of 'derived biotypes'.

There are multiple points of similitude between the two biotypologies.

A synthetic summary is presented in Table 2. It must be borne in mind that other features are more primarily related to oriental medicine and to that specific constitutional typological medicine.

Table 2. Synthesis of old and new biotypology

Traditional Element	Fire	Earth	Water	Air
Hippocratic (450 BC)	Blood	Yellow Bile	Black Bile	Phlegm
Temperament	Hot/dry	Cold/dry	Cold/wet	Hot/wet
Unani (1000AD)[1]	Sanguine (hot/wet)	Choleric (hot/wet)	Melancholic (cold/dry)	Phlegmatic (cold/wet)
Jorjani (1100AD)[2]	Fire (warm/dry)	Soil	Water	Air (warm/wet)
S. Hildegard B. (1200 AD)	Sanguine	Choleric	Melancholic	Phlegmatic
Sigaud (1893)[3]	Muscular	Cerebral	Digestive	Respiratory
SCM (ca 1900AD)	SE	TE	SY	TY
Sheldon (ca 1950 AD)	Mesomorphic		Endomorphic	Exomorphic
TCMC (ca 1970 AD)	Balanced/ Neutral	Phlegm dampness	Qi stagnation	Yang deficient
Dominating hormone Oberhammer (2017)	Adrenaline	Somatotropin	Vasopressin	Cortisol
Ayurveda	Pitta	Kapha	Pitta/Kapha	Vata

(To be continued in the next page)

Traditional Element	Fire	Earth	Water	Air
Tibetan medicine	Mkhris pa	Bad kan	Bad kan	Rlung
Hahnemann (1833)[1]:	Psora		Sycosis	Syphilis
Von Grauvogl (1870)[2]	Psora	Pseudopsora	Sycosis	Syphilis
Endocrine equivalent [4]	Hyperpituitary	Hypersurrenal	Hypothyroidal	Hyposurrenal
Pende (1912)[4]	Long-limbed sthenic	Short-limbed sthenic	Short-limbed asthenic	Long-limbed asthenic
Viola (1909)	Athletic		Pyknic	Asthenic
Mario Barbara (1920)[5]	Normotype		Megalo-splanchnic	Micro-splanchnic
Ernst Kretschmer (1921)	Muscular athletic		Pyknic	Asthenic
Dr. Eric Berg [6] (2015)	Adrenal	Liver	Ovary	Thyroid

1: as exposed by Little (2014, pg. V5 pg. 6-30) to define the miasms
2: as exposed by Rajgurav and Aphale (2016)
3: based on the characteristics explained by Ramos-Jimenex et al. (2016)
4: as exposed by Duvernier 1965
5: as exposed by Stern (2016)
6: as presented in http://www.DrBerg.com.

Also, Ayurveda, not to be confounded with Tibetan medicine as they are two different medical systems, has a concept of body constitution. Differently from the traditional western view of the four humours, and from Tibetan medicine, Ayurveda has three humours and three main body types. Indeed, Ayurveda assigns an individual into one of the seven main constitutive types, or prakriti, based on the inherent imbalance of the three energy forces, or dosha, called Vata, Pitta and Kapha.

This is just an initial tentative systematic review of the somatotypes as elaborated by various medicines and physicians over the centuries. A more detailed and comprehensive synthetic process in this field of science (the convergence of Western and Eastern/Oriental traditions of medicine), would be recommended as the current summary lacks fundamental clarity at this time in history. Further studies are warranted to increase our knowledge of the correspondence of the various biotypes on several levels.

3.5.2.4 *Psychobiological links*

There have been many proposals over the decades to align the four temperaments with the Hippocratic humors.

The main association used throughout the ages has been summarized in Table 3.

Table 3. Standard temperament/humoral association (adapted from Emtiazy et al., 2012; Senior, 2008)

Humor	Phlegm	Blood	Yellow bile	Black bile
Qualities	Cold/wet	Hot/wet	Hot/dry	Cold/dry
Element	Water	Air	Fire	Earth
Temperaments	Phlegmatic	Sanguine	Choleric	Melancholic
Myers-Briggs	SJ	SP	NT	NF

Myers-Briggs Abbreviations: F, feeling; J, judging; N, intuitive; P, perceiving; S, sensing; T, thinking.

Summary by Emtiazy et al. (2012).

The Hippocratic postulation of the four humors, as combined to the four elements (air, fire, water, earth), thought of, in ancient times, to be the constituents of everything, is related both to the concept of humors in Roman times, through Galen and many others, such as the writings of Carl Jung in the early twentieth century, and the Myers-Briggs Type Inventory personality types, still in popular use today, would form the basis of the four-fold characteristics of individual differences.

Throughout the 20th century, different psychologists proposed their own views of the four temperaments. These are:

- Pavlov (1897), who used the humors to describe his dogs' personalities;
- Adickes (1905), who talks about the "Four World Views", namely "innovative," "traditional," "doctrinaire," and "skeptical";
- Spranger (1914), refers to the "Four Value Attitudes" of "artistic," "economic," "religious," and "theoretic";

p. 64/193

- Kretschmer (1920), called them "manic", "depressive", "oversensitive", "insensitive";

- Fromm (1947), four psychological orientations are exploitative, hoarding, receptive, and marketing;

- Eysenck (1947): the first psychologist to use a psycho-statistical method identifying two major dimensions of human personality: (1) Neuroticism (N) and (2) Extraversion (E);

- Pritchard (1952): found a correlation between extroverts' sociability and their oral fluency;

- Myers (1958), refers to humors as "perceiving", "judging", "feeling", "thinking", and modified an earlier theory from Carl Jung;

- Kiersey (1978): divided humans into "idealists", "rationals", "guardians" and "artisans";

- Stern (1983): noticed that extroverts are dominant in obtaining communication skills;

- Littauer (1992): further developed the 4 temperaments in his own brand of phycological types;

- Montgomery (2002), used instead letters "SP", "SJ", "NF", and "NT";

- Ellis (2008): noticed that extroverts were advantaged at acquiring basic interpersonal communicative skills,.

Whether these personality characteristics are dependent on biochemical, biophysical (electromagnetic) and structural/energetic make-up of the persons is yet to be fully demonstrated. But given the interdependent nature of attitudes, its role in biological relationships, this cannot be excluded a priori.

Neurochemical abnormalities were demonstrated relate to genes and to key components of major depression. This indicates that, through biochemical (hormonal) imbalances, the constitution may affect selectively the display of temperaments. The concept of endophenotype is linked to neurophysiological, biochemical, endocrinological, neuroanatomical, cognitive, and neuropsychological structure.

3.5.2.5 *Temperaments*

Since Galen's proposal of the four humors, behavioral scientists have been interested in the creation of various models to integrate physical and psychological factors. An integration of normal personality variation and psychiatric disorders with neurobiological mechanisms, in a unified biosocial theory of personality has been attempted. But Galen did not invent this out of the blue.

No, it seems that these ideas came to our day from the father of modern medicine, Hippocrates himself. In some Hippocratic treatises we already find the idea that bodily fluids are not merely the building blocks of people's physical constitution, but also affect their mental dispositions.

The Four Temperaments theory is one of several behavior-oriented theories that modern psychology has adopted from ancient schools of philosophy. These four temperaments were quickly matched up also to Empedocles' four primary elements (air, water, earth, and fire).

All theories claiming human personality as a function of nature (or heredity), developed by behaviorists, cognitivists, constructivists, and other psychologists during the 20th century, are called temperament theories. And this alone should justify and sustain any claim on the reality of the matter.

Since temperament is an aspect of our personality (a trait or predisposition to display certain behavioral tendencies), it is genetically based, inborn, there from birth or even before. Hence it is forged into the structure of the human body, whether genetic, epigenetic and/or energetic (biochemical and biophysical).

A summary of the psychological traits of similarity with the temperaments throughout a few of the major theories is presented in Table 4.

Table 4. Psychological Theories and the Four Temperaments

Psychological				
Aristoteles (325 BC)	Sensual	Material	Logic	Ethic
Galen (190 AD)	Sanguine	Melancholic	Phlegmatic	Choleric
Paracelsus (1550)	Everchanging	Diligent	Curious	Inspired
Adickes (1905)	Innovator	Traditional	Sceptic	Teacher
Spranger (1914)	Esthetic	Economic	Theoretic	Religious
Kretschemer (1920)	Hypomanic	Depressive	An-aesthetic	Hyper-aesthetic
Fromm (1947)	Explorer	Accumulator	Merchant	Receptive
Meyer (1958)	Pusher	Scheduler	Headstrong	Friendly
Littauer (1992)	Popular	Powerful	Perfect	Peaceful
Montgomery (2002)	SP	SJ	NT	NF
Kiersey (2012)	Artisan	Guardian	Idealist	Rational

p. 68/193

3.6 Conclusions

Any scientific data ever acquired for the confirmation of certain biotypologies, of whatever type of constitutional medicine, apply to and throughout all other constitutional medicine typologies. A confirmation of eastern constitutional medicine automatically confirms western constitutional medicine.

What has become obvious is that a different body structure is the result of a particular hormonal balance (or the other way around). The influence of the entire endocrine system will eventually affect the psychobiology of the individual. The emergence of certain attitudes or temperaments (the psychological traits of an individual's mind) are the result of the body structure and type.

It was shown also how humoral pathology was derived from the observation of the unhealthy blood, in the form of different layers of the blood.

A constitution can be modelled as the sum of an individual's physical build, thinking / processing style and temperament (including reactivity and susceptibility). The main point of interest is not the diversity of classifications, but the fact that these observers (researchers) have described, more or less, the same corresponding types of physique.

It should be noted though that none of these systems of physique identification can apply to serious genetic diseases. The reason is that an external deformity or physiologic malformation is a biological "error" not a normal state of nature.

This will certainly lead us individualized treatment fully emphasizing the individual differences of people based on the various constitutions. This new medicine will formulate individual medical designs and adopt optimal and targeted therapeutic interventions. The optimal treatment program for a particular patient will facilitate the choice for more targeted and appropriate lifestyles, that enhance the health and safety of the patient.

4 A New Medicine

We have by now understood the basic scientific background of the ABO blood typing and the constitutions in ancient medicine. If you haven't read the previous chapter, no worries: it is not a must. There is no need to read it if you are not interested in the scientific proof and evidence of the method. Nor do I recommend it if you are not attracted to this kind of information.

It is time to look at what we can factually do to help integrate these two similar though different worldviews.

A more integrated approach is certainly helpful to view each person in the totality of the biochemical and biophysical possibilities of the human body.

We will be concentrating on the four humours or four temperaments paradigm and on the four ABO blood groupings. We have seen how modern science does recognize these as scientific, undisputable facts (in the previous chapter). Now, we should see how recent research in several fields of scientific study can shed some light on the characteristics of these concepts.

The humoral concept of medicine believes not only that a well-balanced lifestyle yields a healthy mind and body but also enables you to recognize who you are. The ABO blood type diet refers at specific biochemical factors that model the way our body responds to stimuli. But also, wellness is maintained or restored by balancing opposite forces (or humours), such as heat and cold, or dryness and wetness.

Do you start to feel how these two systems of thought are very much interdependent, non-exclusive, and similar, in a certain sense? If not, no worries. It will become clear in a few pages.

The most important thing to remember is that though different we all are, we are also similar in certain degrees. By recognizing the differences and similarities with a couple of classifications we can understand better who we are physically and biologically. Our limits and potentialities will be then unmasked. Once you know them, you will be empowered to do whatever is in your proper constitutional (body's) potential to do.

4.1   Western Body Types

4.1.1 Introduction

It is not surprising that we can think about the following: structural (physical) and constitutive (hormonal and biophysical) substrates talk to each other. Yes, in our body these two forms or characteristics can condition one another.

The physical structure of our body communicates in a bidirectional manner with the biochemical (simply, hormonal) structure of the same body. When I say bidirectional I mean that also the biochemical features of our body communicate with its respective shape and form (and manipulate or influence it).

This occurs in the whole of the body, including its most important organ: the brain. So, the physical and biochemical traits of the body condition will influence the mind to form emergent personality dimensions.

As this has been proposed by many scientists in the past (and also in the present), we shall take advantage of this knowledge. We shall proceed by converging towards a more integrated approach to the topic of biotypes.

While we do this, we should remember a simple truth. To be able to correctly identify body constitutions requires skill and experience. While skill can be learned, experience is something that you have to gain on the ground. Being able to describe constitutions accurately is still a rather undeveloped aspect of modern biomedicine. So, don't worry as we will try to develop a synthetic and easily understandable approach to this problem.

4.1.2 Standard Ancient Constitutions

According to Galen, there are nine possible mixtures (he called them, kraseis) of qualities in the human body. In the first place, there are people whose physical constitution is dominated by one of the four qualities. Secondly, there are four constitutional types that are dominated by a pair of qualities, hot and wet, hot and dry, cold and wet, and cold and dry. The ninth possible krasis (constitution) is a balanced distribution of all four qualities; this is the optimal state of the human body.

This is briefly and graphically shown in Figure 13.

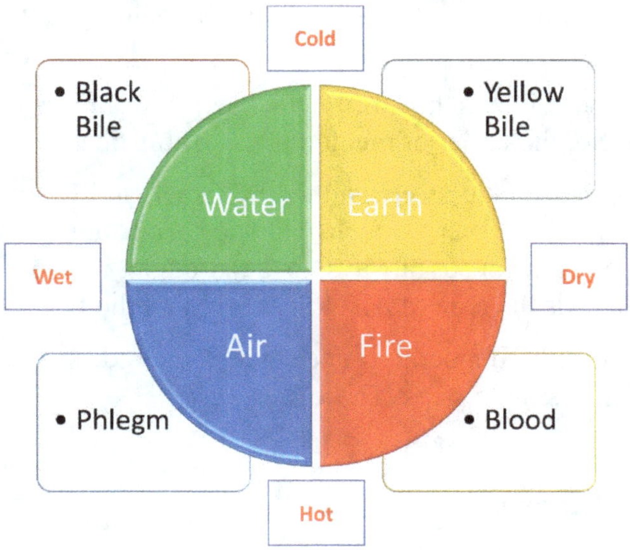

To note, the balanced form is still to be found. That is, we are all unbalanced.

Of course, Galen did not come up with this distinction alone. He brought it from someone else: Hippocrates, the father of medicine. In fact, Hippocrates formulated a set of principles that helped to define the tendencies (i.e., temperaments) of each patient. He defended that the root of one's temperament derived from the four humors dominant in the body. The dominant humor is derived from the pattern of response to environmental forces (e.g., wind, earth, water, and fire) in the following manner:

i.   blood (sanguine, warm, and pleasant);

ii. black bile from the liver (choleric, hot-tempered);

iii. phlegm (phlegmatic, apathetic);

iv. yellow bile from the kidneys (melancholic, depressed, and sad).

In the Hippocratic perspective, disease, though produced by nature, was also cured by nature (nature was seen as the doctor's ally, not the doctor's enemy). So, the physician, unlike the surgeon, served as the handmaiden to nature, not by curing, but by helping nature to heal.

Is this not the case with all holistic medicines? I would say a resounding YES! So, the father of medicine was a holistic guru.

No, seriously. True medicine as envisioned by Greek and Roman masters of this art was very much holistic. And this is a fundamental aspect that needs always to be brought into each healing system. This is the core of ABO-PLUS TM method.

To do this, what did Hippocrates and then Galen do? They developed a series of simple steps. These are:

- Diagnosis
- Integrated Reasoning
- Patient-centered

The first step is the diagnosis of the state of the whole body of the patient. The art of diagnosis is based on observation. It involved, in ancient times, the use of all five senses (sight for the Hippocratic structure; physical palpation, etc.). Physicians were also skilled at comparing between cases and inferring similarities and differences during the diagnosis.

The second step is the use of integrated reasoning. Some writers refer to it as Hippocratic empiricism (be down to earth and try to be materialistic, in a certain sense). According to this, each individual sign or symptom alone may not convey a clear meaning since they are rarely a determining factor. But each symptom should be combined with many other different and likely interdependent factors (patient's lifestyle, other signs, aspects from the history, etc.). It is only at this stage that the physician could generate a unified and interconnected view of the patient, as a whole (thus, holistic).

The third step is the focus is on the patient (whole-body) and not on the disease. It is the patient who has a unique constitution (in both the western and modern sense). We would need to verify its physical (western biotype) and biochemical (ABO blood type) make-up. This is key as various ABO-PLUS^{TM} body types will react differently to the environment and to treatments.

4.1.3 Modern Western Constitutions

We will not simply rest upon the standard form of biotypology as proposed by Hippocrates and Galen as related even later in the same medicinal system. Instead, I will use the more original formulation of the biotypes, as adopted, and exposed by St. Hildegard of Bingen in "Causae et Curae" (Sellerio, 2015).

St. Hildegard of Bingen (1098-1179) was German Benedictine abbess and polymath. She was a writer, composer, philosopher, mystic and visionary prophet (she was called the Sibyl of the Rhine). Not only this but she was also known as a medical writer and practitioner without even having a degree. In her key medical work "Causae et Curae" liber II, book two (Sellerio, 2015, pg. 127-132, 146-149), St. Hildegard of Bingen has re-proposed the traditional view of the four humors and temperaments but has somewhat altered it by:

- considering the four temperaments valid for both men and women; hence has doubled the temperaments as four for men and four for women for a total of 8 temperaments – two quartets (melancholic, choleric, phlegmatic and sanguine) one for men and one for women;

- the two quartets are very similar to one another, having the same base temperament, but are described very differently in both physical and psychological terms – a melancholic man has substantial structural and temperamental/attitudinal differences to a melancholic woman;

- associating the temperaments to different elements thus having sanguine = fire, phlegmatic = air, melancholic = water and choleric = earth;

Similarly, Simona Oberhammer (Oberhammer, 2017) has identified four base types, easily linked to the traditional four elements, to which four master hormones have been associated and has diversified these four biotypes into male and female, thus obtaining a total of 8 base types.

We have thus the base of modern western constitutional medicine as it is evident in Table 5.

Table 5. Modern Western Constitutional Medicine

Traditional Element	Fire	Earth	Water	Air
Hippocratic (450 BC)	Blood	Yellow Bile	Black Bile	Phlegm
Temperament	Hot/dry	Cold/dry	Cold/wet	Hot/wet
Unani (1000AD)[1]	Sanguine (hot/wet)	Choleric (hot/wet)	Melancholic (cold/dry)	Phlegmatic (cold/wet)
S. Hildegard B. (1200AD)	Sanguine	Choleric	Melancholic	Phlegmatic
Contemporary	Red	Yellow	Green	Blue

4.2 ABO as constitutional medicine

4.2.1 What is ABO Blood Group

We have seen how the four humors can produce four distinct body types. This is evident from the physical structure of human body itself, firstly, and then from the derived biological diversity. There is another division that is purely biochemical. This is the ABO blood grouping.

We cannot see it visually as for the western body types. This division of humanity is internal. So, without the advent of modern technology we would not have guessed about this differential description of chemical and biological behavior of the human body. Nor even understood it.

We now can quickly identify the blood type of each individual with simple diagnostic kits easily available in the market and at a very low cost. Once that is done we can then classify him or her (or ourselves) in one of the four blood types.

The concept of ABO constitutions is the direct result of the difference between people of diverse blood types. It is known that ABO group are determined by glycans (very small carbohydrates). Glycans are like tiny pieces of fibers (non-digestible carbohydrates). These tiny pieces are normally seen at the end of certain carbohydrates present in our body. Whether long or short, they are at the ending part (that part which is exposed to the external environment). These glycans are then called ABO determinants (since they are determined or defined by them) or antigens. Big names, but really nothing that complicated. An antigen is a molecule (with a defined molecular structure) that can stimulate an immune response. And this is the reason for the existence of blood types.

But you might ask, why are they called blood types? They are called blood group (or type) antigens (determinants) because they were found in the blood. But that's not where they are solely. Indeed, they are in many places in the human body.

There are 4 blood groups but only three antigens (or glycans) at the end of each carbohydrate. The three glycans are called A, B and O. So, there are three groups (A, B and O), with one additional group having both A and B glycans, together. This last group is the AB group.

The ABO blood group glycans are present on ALL human cells and tissues. I repeat, ALL human cells and tissues. Yes, you read it right. This is not an insignificant or inconsequential thing. Let's think about it for a moment. If these are present on the membranes of all human cells, then they could potentially interact with anything in the environment surrounding our cells.

And that's exactly what happens.

4.2.2 Why are Blood Groups so Important?

The ABO blood type is a determining factor in several biological events. It is deemed to be a key biochemical characteristic of an individual. Being on the top of the membrane of every cell, these small carbohydrates (more like fibers) have peculiar properties that make them unique.

As we said earlier, ABO determinants are rightly also called antigen, as they can provoke an immune response. So, they react with the other proteins and molecules surrounding them in very precise ways. If they are distinct (4 unique blood groups) then they will react differently. That's it: it's that simple.

But that's not the whole story. There's more. The ABO group determinants "star" (i.e., to "be present" on top of) all proteins and fats on the cell membrane and inside the cell. These ABO starred proteins and fats are known as glycoconjugates (big word to say that they are linked to sugars [glyco]). Now, these glycoconjugates are not just on the membrane of cells but are also found in the plasma and in various other body fluids and secretions. Yes, even in the biological fluids of the body, anywhere proteins and fats are free to move.

To make the long story short. They are practically everywhere.

Being everywhere, their likeliness to interfere with all normal processes is extremely high. For example, they are found on glycolipids (fats with carbohydrate structures linked to them) and glycoproteins of the mucous layer of the gastrointestinal tract. The function of mucous layer is to protect and cover the internal tissues of the gastrointestinal tract. The stomach and the gut in general are covered by a mucous layer. Guess what? They are present here too.

p. 78/193

What this means in simple and direct terms is that they are in contact with the food that we ingest. In direct contact. As soon as we ingest any food, the ABO blood group glycans will find themselves in close proximity with food molecules. And they will likely react in one way or another with these.

ABO blood group glycans are linked to specialized biomolecular interactions between cells and other cells or other freely circulating biomolecules (biological molecules). Moreover, the same types of interactions occur between cells and microbes. The bugs that are in our intestine react too to the various glycans. The intestinal bugs are known as resident microbiota (or microflora), meaning that they reside there normally. These bugs (being non-human cells) have glycans too and have ways to recognize glycans.

Do you start to see how and why the ABO blood group glycans are becoming so significant?

They are everywhere, especially on cells.

They react with almost everything, especially certain proteins.

They react with food molecules as they become in close contact with them.

Cells of the intestine react with microbial cells also through their interaction (ABO blood group antigens). Hence…

They react also with the gut microflora.

The game is set!

But there's more.

4.2.3 The Holobiont blood group

We have just seen that ABO blood groups are present on cells of the gut that react with microbial cells (bugs). They don't just react passively to the presence of bugs. Not at all. They react actively: they define the microbiological structure of the gut. That is, they define which bugs can reside and which should not. There is a clear connection between the blood grouping and the composition of microbial communities within the human body.

And not just in the gut. Please don't be shocked by this affirmation. We don't have bugs in the belly. They're everywhere. Yes, absolutely. Everywhere in our body we can and in fact do find bugs. And they, the bugs, are not harmful. On the contrary. They are like helpers.

I know. I am telling you something that is odd, to say the least. But it is just and simply the truth. Bugs are everywhere within us, and they are living harmoniously with us and within us. These bugs are called symbionts, that is, collaborators. We help them and they help us. How do we help them? By providing them a niche (a place to live) and food. Yes, we give them food to eat. I will explain but first let's see what they give us back.

The bugs have a different genetic make-up with respect to us. Having different genes, they make diverse proteins and enzymes. And this is the point. They have much more enzymes that what we humans have. And this brings about a second key concept. We are physically the sum of all the cells in our body. Of all species.

Boom!

Yes, of all species. We ARE the SUM of all species present in our body. And numerically they (the bugs) vastly outnumber our human cells. I mean, they are smaller but more numerous.

I know, this is a shocker!

We, as humans are considered as holobionts. Holobionts are a mixture of various organisms belonging to thousands of different species. As holobionts we have the genetic capacity of the sum of all the diverse species living in us. If you go on the net and type in "holobiont" you will be amazed.

Now, back to where we were.

The ABO (together with other glycans, Lewis etc. [not important]) glycans expressed in the GI tract seem to actually shape the

p. 80/193

composition of gut microbiota. How? As we said earlier, by providing the right type of nutrients for certain specific bacterial species and families.

It is known that glycans (being essentially undigestible carbohydrates) are used as food sources by those microbes with the appropriate toolkit to digest them. The right toolkit is intended in terms of a specified set of enzymes defined genetically by the microorganism. Therefore, the blood type grouping is selective to certain microorganisms who will in the end shape the composition of the gut microflora.

And not just in the intestinal microflora, but also the microbiota in every tissue of the human body. There are millions of ecological niche in the human body, each with its own resident microbes (i.e., living normally or thriving). And this is selected by the blood group.

We can then conclude that each blood group has its own specific microbiome. And because of the specificity of the microflora, the bugs in turn confer particular enzymatic capabilities to the host (us humans). So, a select host with, say, an A blood type will have a microbiota that is different from that other hosts of diverse blood groups. And this host (A blood type) will consequently have different enzymatic capacities with respect to a B blood type or O, etc.

The peculiar enzymatic capacity then translates into a physical characteristic of the person being able to digest better certain foods and not others. And if digestion is related to absorption and utilization, then the circle is closed. Based on one's blood type, an individual can digest absorb and simply utilize better certain foods and not others.

And this peculiar enzymatic capacity coupled with the ABO glycans on proteins and fats is involved in practically every interaction of your body. This does not just manifest itself in a distinct diet but also in distinctive reactions to diseases and health.

The ABO group thus forms a division of humanity in constitutions or biotypes, where each biotype reacts in its own way to stimuli.

The diversity does not have to be markedly different. For example, I am not saying that a man of a specific blood type becomes blue when he runs. Obviously, not. That is not the case. What I and many other scientists are saying is that the human responses are within a biologically comprehensible range. Within this range, some people are at the center, others are close to the limit. In some of these biological responses, the blood type is a fundamental factor.

We can say that the ABO constitutions are associated at least to a certain degree with susceptibility to disease. And this is described extensively by all ancient medical traditions, even though they knew nothing about blood types. But their knowledge and experience helped them to draw a link between constitutions and disease susceptibility.

4.2.4 Consequences

A normal state of health is defined by an equilibrium between all processes, good and bad bugs (with good prevailing, evidently) and all systems within the holobiont. It is only when the equilibrium is broken that we have illness in one form or another.

This is in line with the standard interpretation of Western and Eastern traditional medicine. All ancient medicine considers the best state of equilibrium as the perfect health condition. Hence, one can honestly conclude that when our bugs are in equilibrium, wherever they are in our body, then we are healthy. When, on the other hand, there is a disequilibrium in the normal composition of the microflora, anywhere in the body, we will have an illness.

In this sense, ABO blood glycans do not simply recognize and influence resident bacteria but have the potential to favor all non-pathogenic (allowing them to thrive) bugs. This includes viruses too. Yes, viruses are deemed microorganisms that infect not just us (human cells) but also bacteria (non-human cells). When a virus infects non-eukaryotic (human) cells they are called phages (or bacteriophages). Viruses too are gifted with property differentially recognizing blood type glycans displayed on cells. Consequently, certain viruses can attack preferentially an individual depending on their blood type. This has been shown in various clinical studies. As specific viruses can bind differentially to ABO blood type glycans, so can bacteriophages recognize the same and bind to them with their capsid proteins.

As there are good and bad bugs, there are also good and bad viruses. We normally have trillions of good viruses within us in any single moment of our life. When a virus affects a bacterium, then this will not attack our human cells.

Conversely, ABO blood group antigens or determinants tend to influence pathogenic (bad) microorganisms by forcing them to stay away from the habitat. They make the habitat inhospitable to bad bugs. Nevertheless, bad bugs are always present in very small amounts and can take control if the conditions are right for them. And when they are right for the bad guys, they are wrong for us. A few of these bad conditions include unhealthy food, wrong food for our blood type, stressors of any kind (environmental, chemical, biological), etc.

ABO blood type glycans do not just influence the physical side of the holobiont. These tiny carbohydrates also can affect the psychological side, like all constitutions confirm. The correlation between blood groups and personality have been investigated back in the 1960s. Among the historical approaches to the study of psychological genetics, one of the most interesting was that which seeks to associate a behavioral trait with a somatic trait like a physical feature known to be genetically determined.

In the end, blood grouping is genetically defined by the creation of appropriate enzymes that can rearrange certain very common carbohydrate structures to form the ABO glycans. Thus, constitution and ABO groups are genetically defined. It can really be said that the definition of these glycans is constitutional (linked to the body shape). So, the blood grouping is opens the gates to another form of constitutional medicine that has developed over the past 30 or 40 years around the world.

4.3 Model-Creation

The base form that was chose for the new model is the "matrix".

The matrix has different meanings depending on the field of study; however I will just focus on the only definition which has been mostly used.

Most simply, a mathematical matrix is a set of numbers or symbols (or any other thing), arranged in rows and columns. That's it.

Let's not be scared about the word mathematical. It is actually simpler than you think. And no, we really are not talking about math here. We don't need to understand really anything else. Rows and columns are like those present in a table or in an excel file.

So, if I make up a table and put the ABO groups on a row and the ancient humours on the columns… There it is. It's done. You got it. By the way, you could also do the opposite. It doesn't really matter. The result is the same as in Table 6.

Table 6. ABO-PLUS ^{TM} Matrix

Constitutions	Air	Water	Earth	Fire
A	Air A	Water A	Earth A	Fire A
B	Air B	Water B	Earth B	Fire B
AB	Air AB	Water AB	Earth AB	Fire AB
O	Air O	Water O	Earth O	Fire O

As you can see, the base matrix for the ABO-PLUS™ biotypes is easily represented in a table. The columns correspond to the four basic elements of ancient western biotypology (Air, Water, Earth, and Fire) while rows relate to the four ABO constitutions (blood groups A, B, O and AB).

This base matrix is the foundation of all ABO-PLUS™ biotypology and the understanding of its core. It is our starting point.

What this 4x4 (four by four) matrix is really saying is that among the possible combinations of humans there are 16 clearly identifiable subtypes. Indeed 4 times 4 is 16.

So, each person on the Earth can be described as being placed in one of the orange cells in the center of the table.

This system of classification tells us immediately that though different, we are all similar in a number of characteristics. But through these differences and similarities ABO-PLUS™ can deeply understand each individual physically and biologically. ABO-PLUS™ can reveal the limits and potentialities of each person. Once this is done, you will be encouraged to decide for yourself your future based on your proper constitutional (body-type) potential and personal goals.

5 The ABO-Plus biotype Model

5.1 The Synthesis

It is true that the internal organ structure in Sasang Constitutional Medicine (SCM) is a seesaw model. This can be seen in the SE and SY types as the spleen-kidney seesaw, where the spleen controls the intake of food and the kidney controls the discharge of waste products, and the seesaw model that can be seen in the TE and TY types is the lung-liver seesaw, where the lung controls the consumption of qi and fluid and the liver controls the storage of qi and fluid, so it is also true that the physiological and pathological features of each constitution are determined by hyperactive and hypoactive states of visceral groups that are believed to be intrinsic and congenital. In particular, the authors have described the features of each of the four constitutive types as follows:

a) SE type individuals have a hypoactive spleen group that leads to poor management of food intake and digestion (e.g., digestive malfunctions such as chronic indigestion);

b) SY type has a tendency of hypoactive kidney group, i.e., a weak capacity of waste discharge (such as constipation and disorders related to urinary system like cystitis and renal diseases);

c) TY type is characterized by a hyperactive lung group and a hypoactive liver group that is regarded to be a state of higher catabolism than anabolism (high basal metabolic rate – BMR – and low urination is the main functional shortcoming);

d) TE type's physiological features, being opposite to a TY type, may be equal to an anabolism-dominant state, which may lead to low BMR and a tendency to be overweight.

These attributes tally very well with the biotypes advanced by western thought, and in particular with those exposed and utilized by Oberhammer (2017).

In Sasang constitutional medicine (SCM), Je Ma Lee in 1894 included four of the five body types described in the Yellow Emperor's Inner Classic of Oriental Medicine (Greater Yang type, Lesser Yang type, Greater Yin type, and Lesser Yin type), as the Yin–Yang balanced type (shown in Figure 14), which was described as a perfect human type, did not exist (Kim and Pham, 2011).

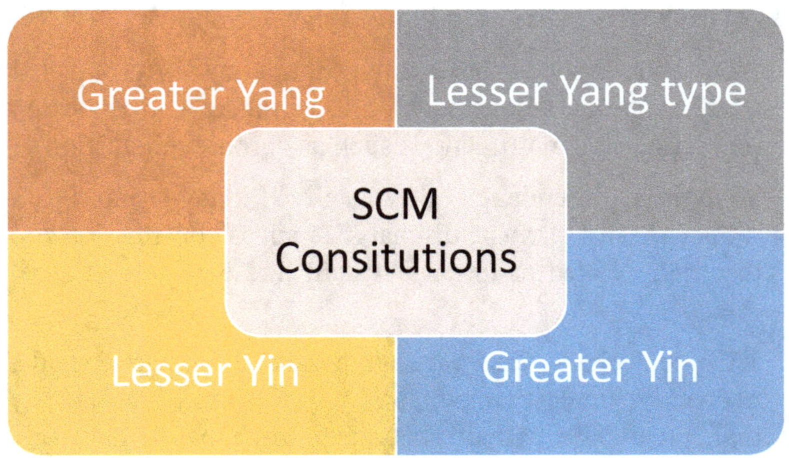

Indeed, if you see how this Figure is reminiscent of the aforementioned four temperaments: then you got it. The similarity is striking. I am not saying that someone copied someone else. No! What I am hinting is that there is an underlying layer of common interpretation between the practitioners of the various ancient and traditional medicines. Four base types.

From this we can now build a framework to put together the two different biotypologies into a single system. But first let's look at the other constitution or biotypology. The blood typology.

5.2   Introduction

Constitution represents a physical disposition to be "something". Temperaments are a psychological tendency to manifest emotions in an almost predetermined manner. It is not an inflexible circuitry imprinted in our minds and bodies that inevitably fixates in modes of action-response in us but rather a privileged way manifestation of ideas and emotions. As the biotype may have diverse hormonal concentrations, then better clarified this point when noting that hormones influence three systems (sensory, central nervous, and effectors), so that specific stimuli are more likely to elicit certain responses in the appropriate behavioral or social context.

The very many differences in both hormonal, anatomical (body shape and form) and psychological, behavioral, and neurobiological features have been demonstrated scientifically, for centuries.

With that said, I will now elaborate on a new synthesis of biotypology called 'ABO biotype'.

Because the ABO characteristic is constitutionally dependent on the expression of the ABO group, this is one other constitutional type. Indeed, in terms of both pathogenesis and pathology, human beings differ in their susceptibility to pathogenic factors and their tendencies to progress to disease states. Plenty of clinical trials have demonstrated the differential susceptibility of the various ABO groups towards diseases and pathogens.

By leveraging on the physiologic differences in blood grouping ABO, with four distinct types, A, B, AB, and O, as noticed and confirmed by Mozzi (2012), and merging this with the age-old four elemental constitutions, as synthesized by St. Hildegard (Sellerio, 2015) and Oberhammer (2017), it is possible to divide humankind as in Table 7.

Table 7. ABO constitutional biotypology

HUMANKIND							
AIR		WATER		EARTH		FIRE	
Female	Male	Female	Male	Female	Male	Female	Male
A	A	A	A	A	A	A	A
B	B	B	B	B	B	B	B
AB	AB	AB	AB	AB	AB	AB	AB
O	O	O	O	O	O	O	O

Humans can be divided into 4 basic groups.

Table 7 explicates the division of humankind into four basic constitutive types, which become eight when considering the natural division of sexes and finally multiplied by four ABO types for a total of thirty-two ABO constitutive types. Thus, the first one in the table would be defined as Air (the basic biotype), Female (the sex) with blood type A (conventionally defined as AFA), the last one as Fire, Male and O (conventionally FMO). And so on and so forth.

Temperaments that result from these are, as proposed by Jorjani, either single or pure temperaments (4) or combined (other 4).

Each of these have very specific and distinct from others physiochemical reactivities that make them unique. It would be very interesting in the future to explore the medical features of each individual outlined in Table 7.

5.3   The Physical Structure

5.3.1 General Qualities

Having illustrated the doctrine of the four humors and the basic principles of western medicine, it is now time to define the four constitutions that shall be adopted as a basis for any future analysis.

The bodily constitutions of Galen are mixtures (krasis, temperaments) of the basic qualities (hot, cold, wet, and dry), and the humors (blood, phlegm, yellow bile, and black bile) and is central to any traditional account of health and disease. As for other constitution-based medicines, the number of temperaments or body types may vary depending on several factors (including practitioner's preference, tradition, etc.).

Notwithstanding this, the choice will depend much more on tradition and on the expertise of some renown source.

For these reasons, the source of the biotypes with their explanation and characteristics has been chosen in Medieval times in which period the ancient writers were followed most accurately. The choice fell onto the most gifted expert of traditional Greek and Roman medicine in Medieval Europe: St. Hildegard of Bingen. Writer, scientist, mystic, painter, musician, artist, prominent preacher, composer, healer and nun, Hildegard was an extraordinary woman and is credited of being among the greatest intellectuals the world has ever seen (Menapace, 2019b). She further developed the doctrine of temperaments in her two main scientific writings, "Physica" (Natural History) and "Causae et Curae" (Causes and Cures), which also describes human physiology, psychology and processes of health and disease.

In Causae et Curae (Hildegard, 1999), she delineates four types of men and women according to the one prevailing humour in the body which consequently defined the physiologic and psychologic essence of that biotype. These are shown hereafter.

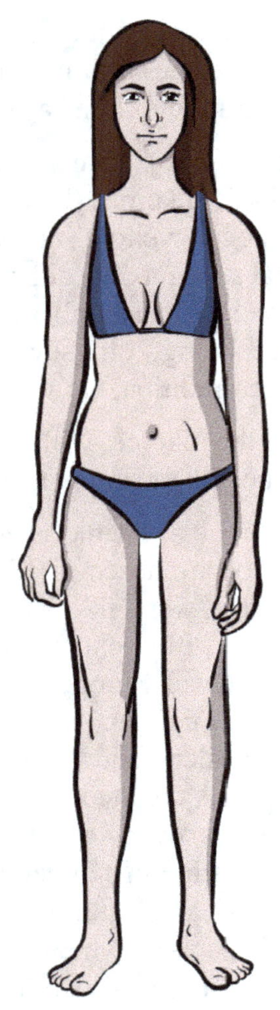

Figure 15. Woman Air Biotype

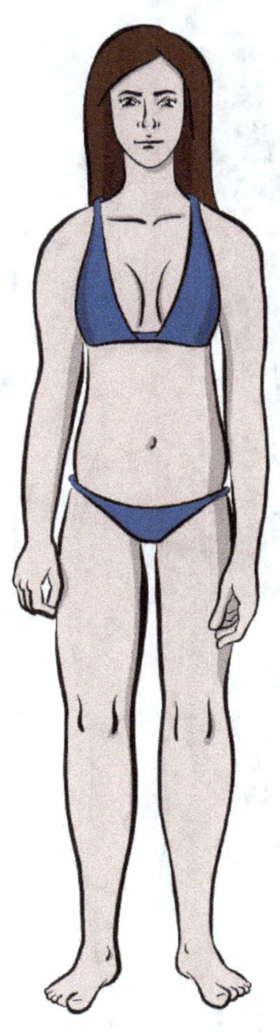

Figure 16. Woman Air Biotype Overweight

Figure 17. Woman Water Biotype

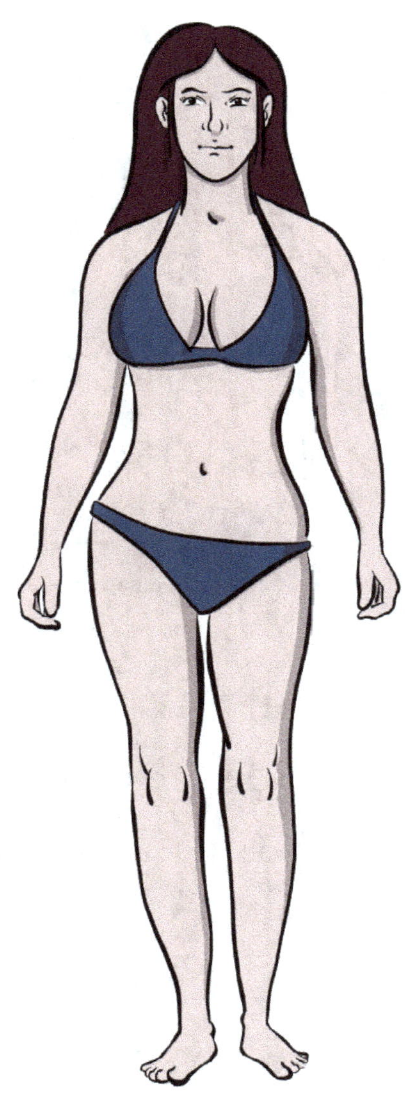

p. 94/193

Figure 18. Woman Water Biotype Overweight

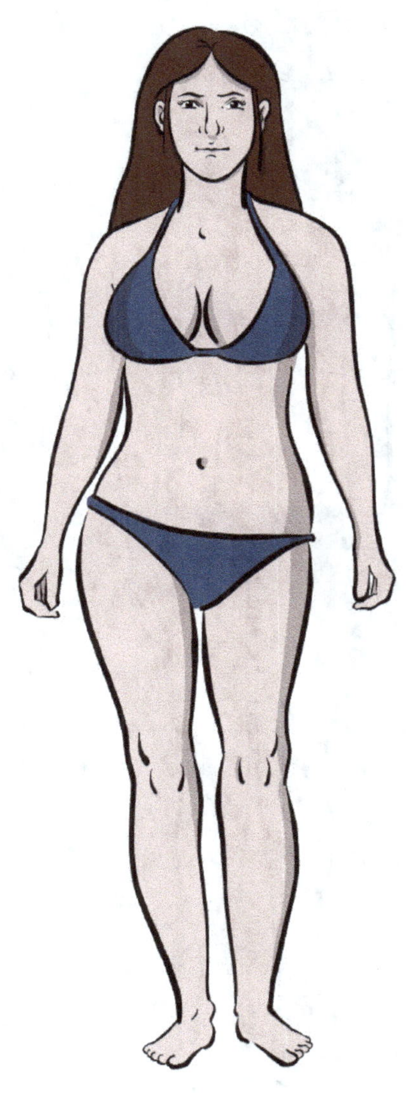

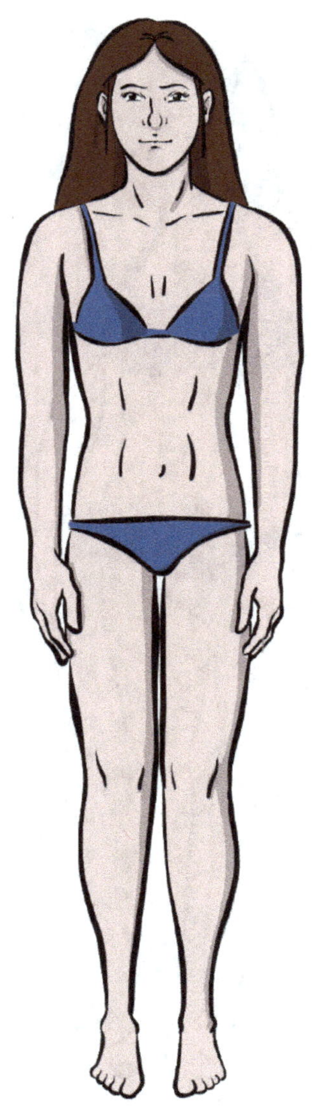

Figure 20. Woman Earth Biotype Overweight

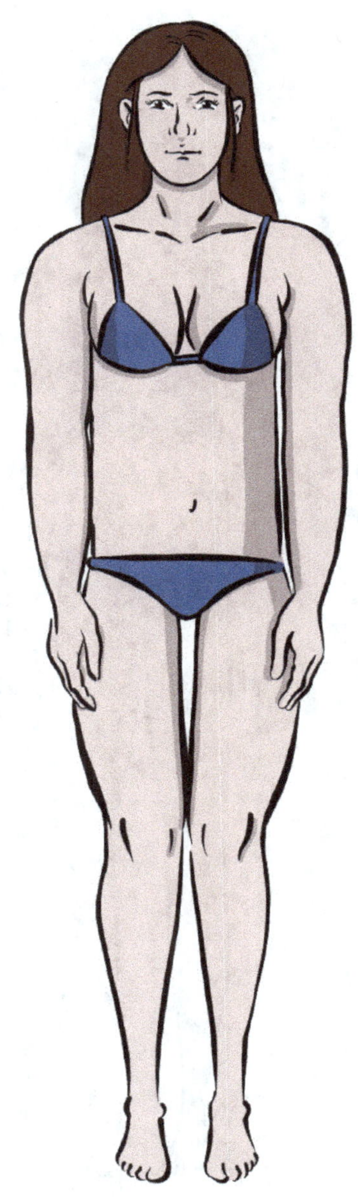

Figure 21. Woman Fire Biotype

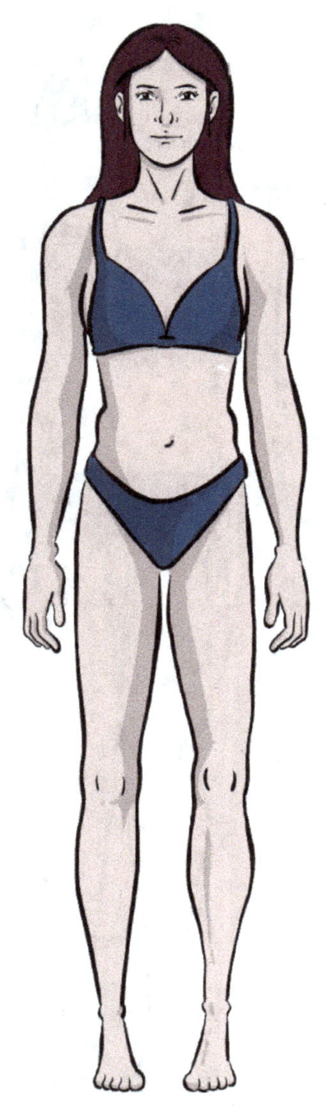

Figure 22. Woman Fire Overweight

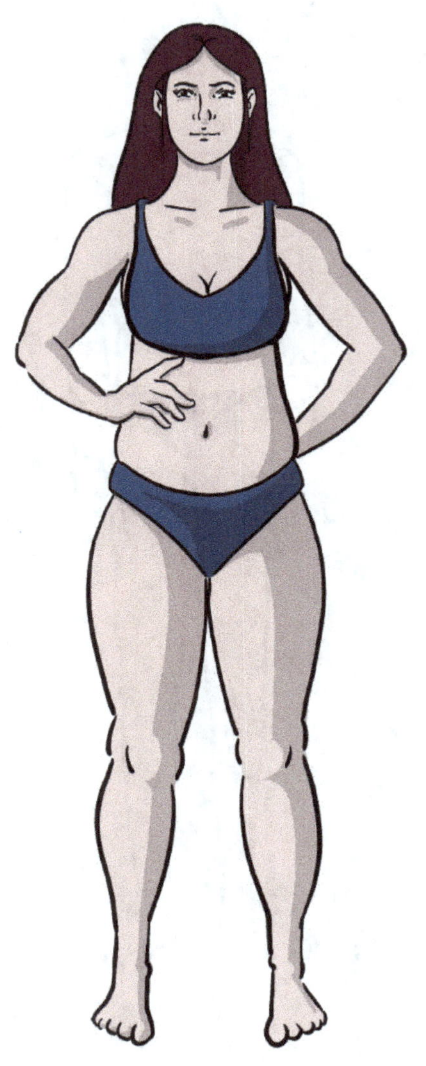

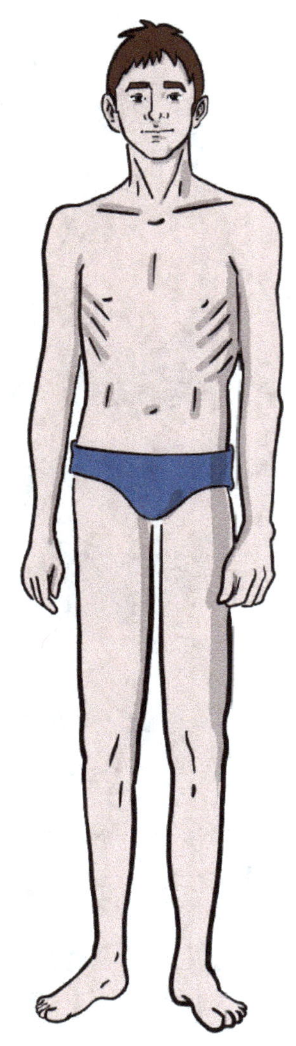

Figure 23. Man Air Biotype

Figure 24. Man Air Biotype Overweight

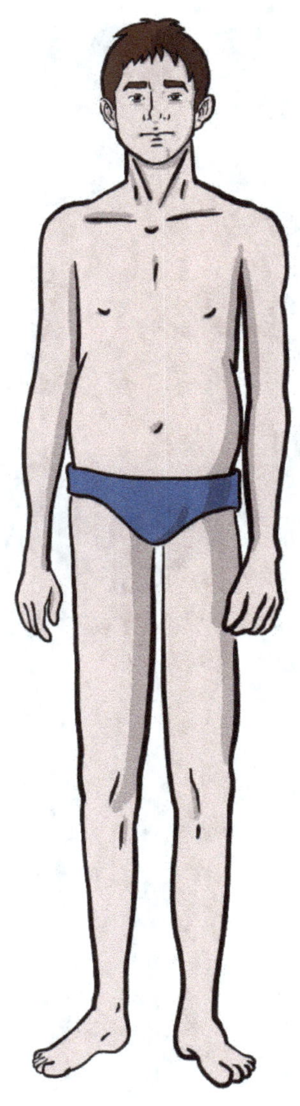

Figure 25. Man Water Biotype

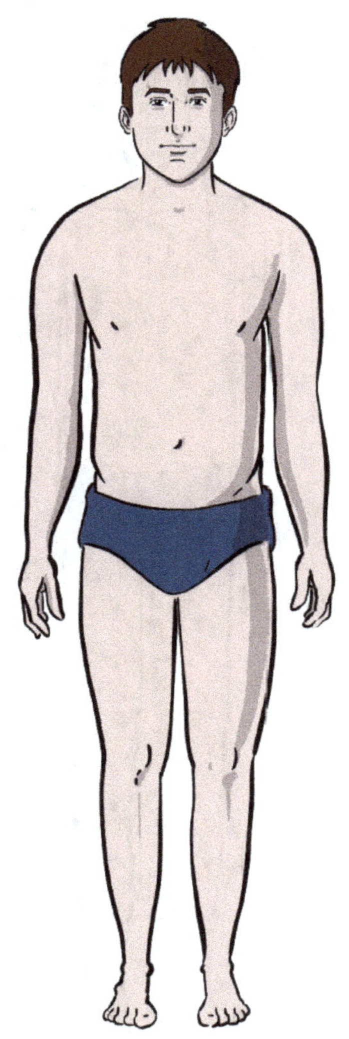

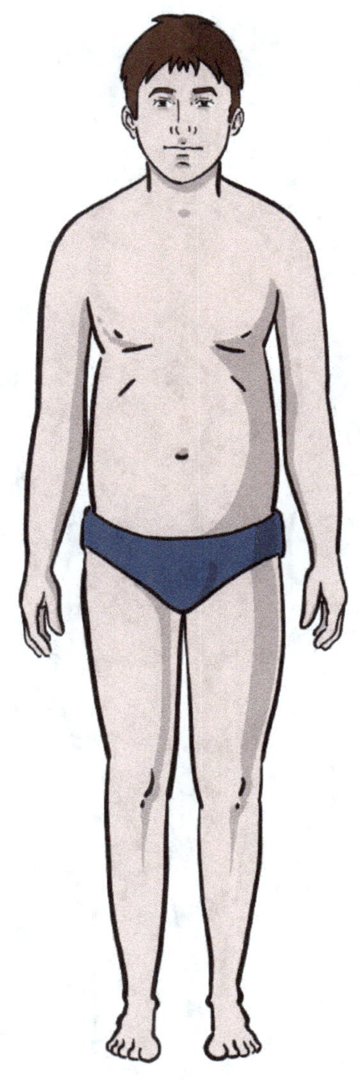

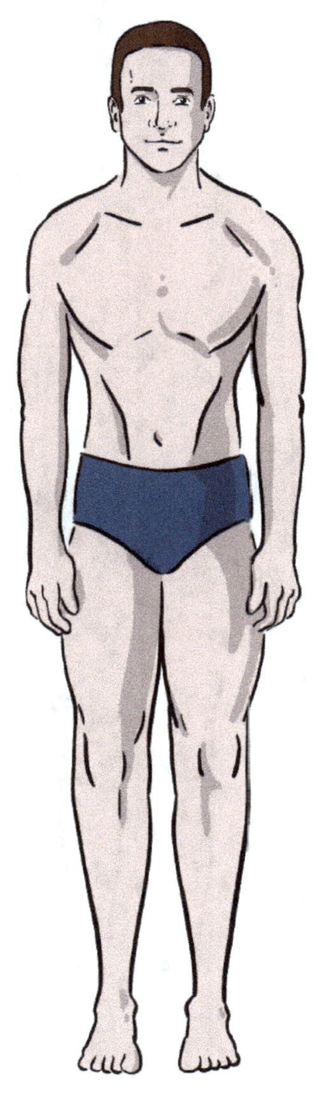

Figure 27. Man Earth Biotype

Figure 28. Man Earth Biotype Overweight

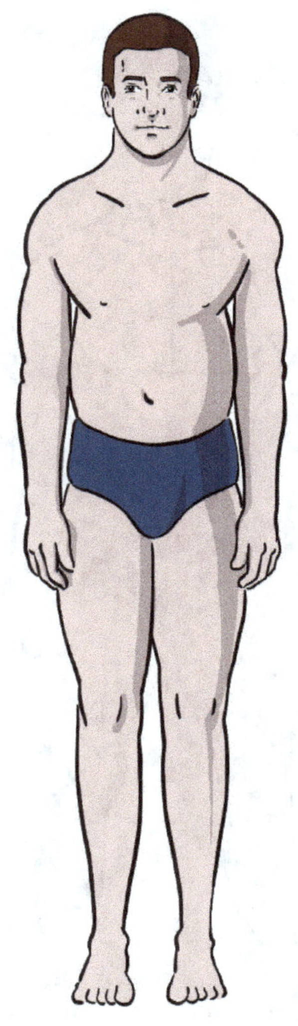

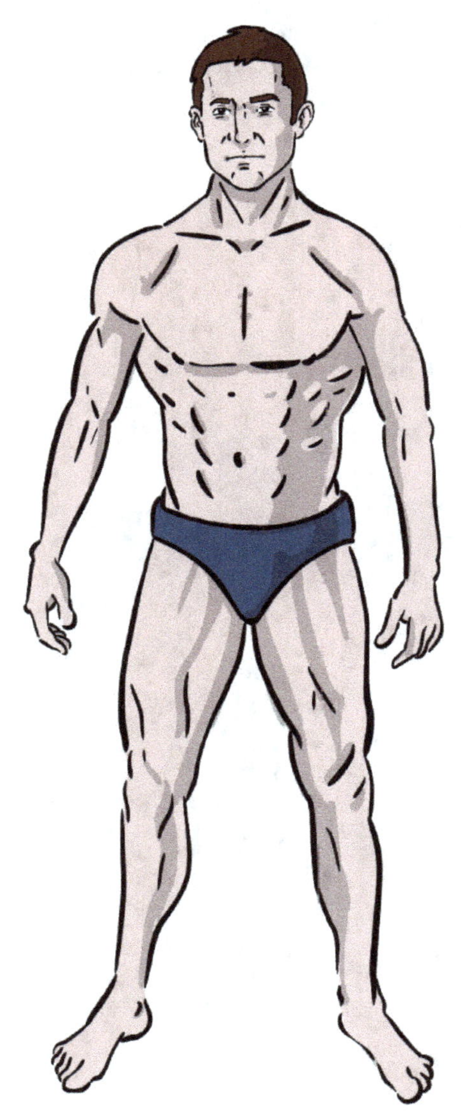

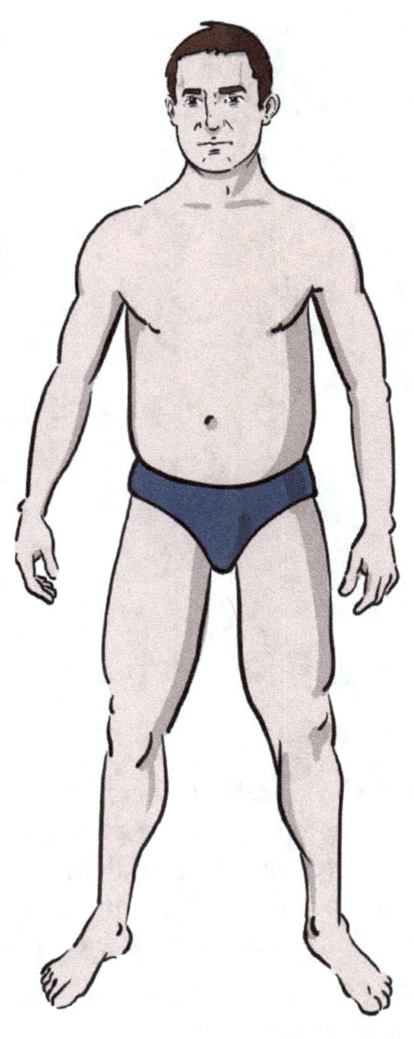

5.3.2 Air biotype

Figure 31. Air biotype physical structure

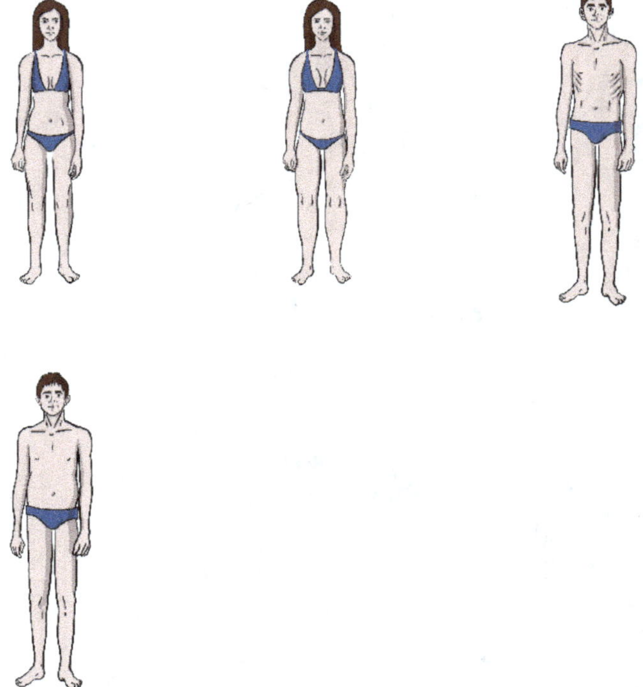

The air biotype has specific air-related characteristics make him or her easily identifiable. Air represents the gaseous state of matter which has as main property that of being light-weighted. Indeed, absence of mass or resistance to accumulation of mass in the form of fat or muscle is the principal characteristic of this biotype.

All other physical traits come as a result of this. Thin bone structure (the thinnest of all biotypes) is the key feature that models the rest of the body. Having this thin bone structure, it is not simple/ possible to build up mass or fat as all the other biotypes can. Further traits are discussed in Table 8.

p. 108/193

Table 8. Main Air Biotype Traits

Hormone	Energy Type	Body Shape	Body Temp
Cortisol	Short, vital	Long, skinny [a]	Cold [b]
Chin	**Neck**	**Head**	**Hand**
Short, thin	Skinny	Dolicocephalic [c]	Long, skinny
Shoulders	**Muscles**	**Skin Type**	**Bone Shape**
Narrow, small	Tonic, thin	Thin, dry	Hypoplastic [d]

a = essentially a thin body type
b = depending on the seasons, can feel hot or cold
c = smaller than other biotypes
d = less developed than other biotypes

5.3.3 Water biotype

Figure 32. Water biotype physical structure

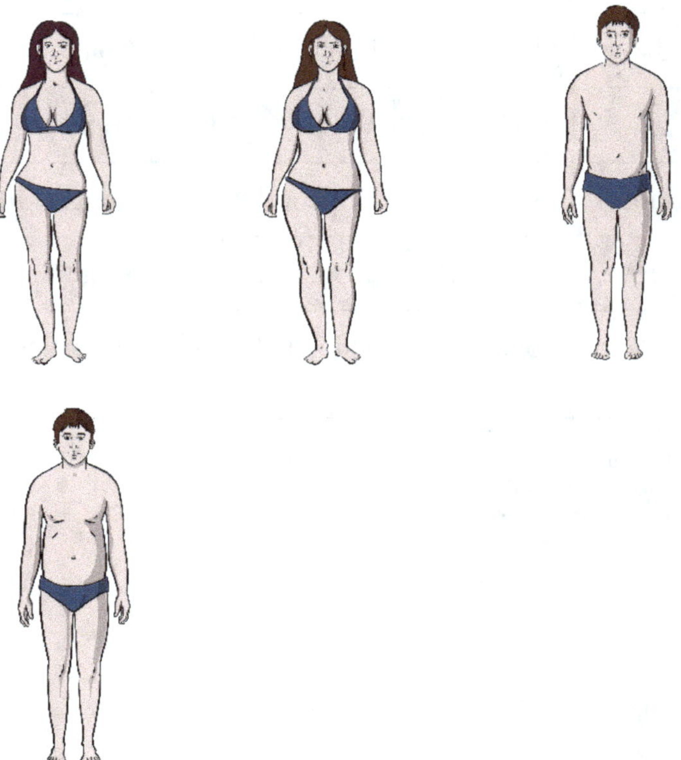

The water biotype has specific water-related characteristics make him or her easily identifiable. Water represents the aqueous/liquid state of matter which has as main property that of being shape-free that is to take the shape of its container. Certainly, this is true for this biotype since water is the main component of the visible mass of the body. Water confers a sense of softness to the body. When in the process of building up fat, the first thing that occurs is an excessive retention of water.

All other physical traits come as a result of this. The bone structure is not much developed (could be seen as thin) and this reflects on

p. 110/193

the final strength and resistance of the body type. Both male and female individuals tend to accumulate water frequently and quickly more than muscle mass.

Further traits are discussed in Table 9.

Table 9. Main Water Biotype Traits

Hormone	Energy Type	Body Shape	Body Temp
Vasopressin	Calm, quiet [a]	Soft, round [b]	Cold
Chin	**Neck**	**Head**	**Hand**
Round, large	Large, not too big	Medium size	Large, soft [c]
Shoulders	**Muscles**	**Skin Type**	**Bone Shape**
Normal, falling	Atonic, thin [d]	Thick but soft	Weak

a = need to rest
b = tends to more curved than other biotypes due to water
c = lack of developed muscle mass
d = atonic means without a big muscle mass

p. 111/193

5.3.4 Earth biotype

Figure 33. Earth biotype physical structure

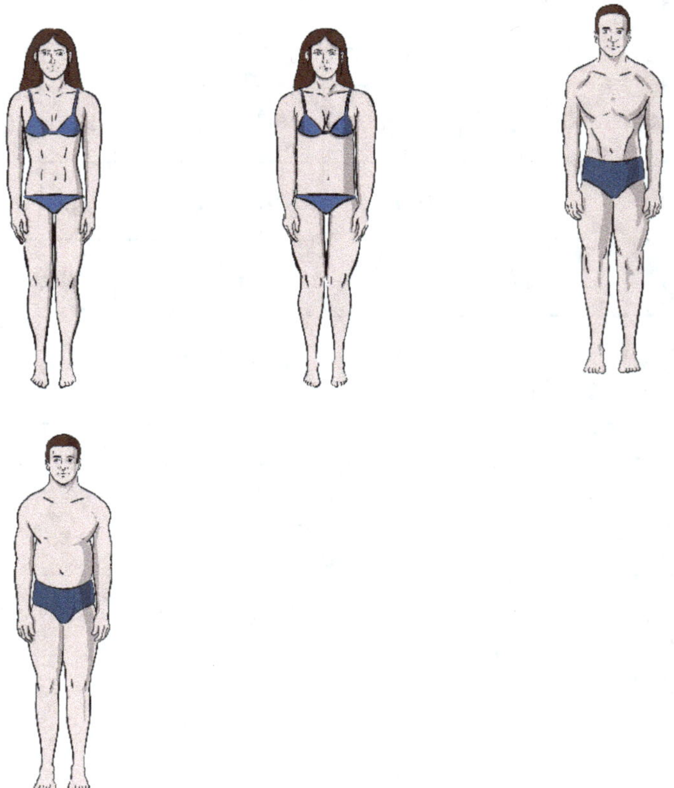

The earth biotype has specific earth-related characteristics make him or her easily identifiable. Earth represents the solid state of matter which has as main property that of being strong, sturdy, and resilient. Earth represents the robustness of the body mass and can withstand long energy expenditures. Earth confers a sense of hardness to the body. The huge muscle mass is normally imbalance, and the bulk of the mass can be found in the upper half of the body.

All other physical traits come as a result of this. The bone structure is very much developed (thick) and this reflects on the final strength and resistance of the body type. Both male and female individuals tend to accumulate fat frequently and quickly more than muscle mass if not cautiously prevented. This is the body builder type.

Further traits are discussed in Table 10.

Table 10. Main Earth Biotype Traits

Hormone	Energy Type	Body Shape	Body Temp
Somatotropin	Resilient [a]	Robust [b]	Warm to hot
Chin	**Neck**	**Head**	**Hand**
Squared, prominent	Large, robust	Large and tall	Large, muscular [c]
Shoulders	**Muscles**	**Skin Type**	**Bone Shape**
Large, oblique	Developed, tonic [d]	Thick and consistent	Robust

a = can resist more than other during work
b = Earth is strong but unbalanced (upper half is larger)
c = large and well-developed muscle mass
d = abundant and big muscle mass

5.3.5 Fire biotype

Figure 34. Fire biotype physical structure

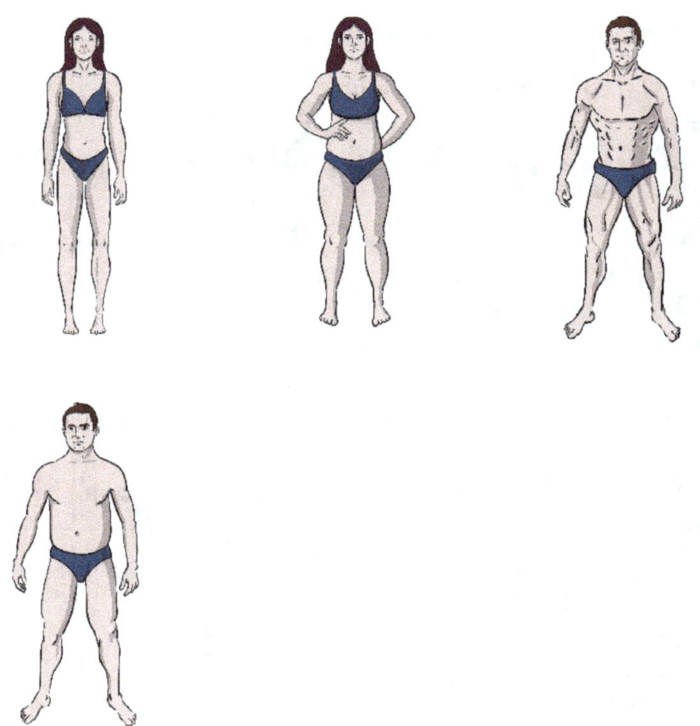

The fire biotype has specific fire-related characteristics make him or her easily identifiable. Fire represents the "plasma" state of matter which has as main property that of light, strong and hot. Fire represents the athletic structure of the body mass and is best shown in balanced body muscles (both upper and lower body well developed). Fire confers a sense of prowess to the body. The structure is designed to achieve resistance in running (and other speed related athletic feats).

All other physical traits come as a result of this. The bone structure is developed (right amount) and this reflects on the final speed and resistance of the body type. Both male and female individuals tend

p. 114/193

to accumulate fat frequently and quickly more than muscle mass if not cautiously prevented. This is the typical athlete.

Further traits are discussed in Table 11.

Table 11. Main Fire Biotype Traits

Hormone	Energy Type	Body Shape	Body Temp
Adrenaline	Constant, Speed [a]	Athletic [b]	Hot
Chin	**Neck**	**Head**	**Hand**
Evident, marked	Long muscular	Well-developed	Long, muscular [c]
Shoulders	**Muscles**	**Skin Type**	**Bone Shape**
Large, straight	Developed, tonic [d]	Consistent, red	Strong

a = burns quickly but lasts quite a long time
b = Fire is strong but balanced
c = well-developed muscle mass in a long hand
d = harmonious muscle mass (athletic)

5.4   An ABO-Plus Example

The two identified biotypologies (ABO and Western Medicine) are not mutually exclusive and have been merged into a matrix. It has been recently shown that an appropriate matrix can be successfully created (Menapace, 2020c). This matrix allows a practitioner to experimentally define a patient.

This formulation of the system (ABO-Plus) allows to take advantage of both the constitutional insights, diagnose diseases and prepare appropriate therapies (dietary recommendations taken from the two forms of medicines, together). An example is shown in Table 12 to aid the process of typification (or as Sheldon taught us somatotyping).

Table 12. Some Characteristics of Individuals AMA and FFO

Characteristics	Source	AMA	FFO
Biological strength	WCM	Weak	Strong
Muscular structure	WCM	Thin (ectomorph)	Well-built (mesomorph)
Metabolism	ABO	Slow	Fast
Predisposition (sports)	ABO	Light training	Hard training
Diet type	WCM	Moist regimen	Dry regimen
Diet type	ABO	Mainly vegetarian	Mostly carnivore
Psychological trait	ABO	Tends to be relaxed	Tends to be active
Psychological trait	WCM	Over-thinker (cerebrotonic)	Action driven (somotomic)

This is an example, and it is not meant to be exhaustive but just typifying.
WCM = western constitutional medicine
AMA = Air, Male, blood type A
FFO = Fire, Female, blood type O

The example of Table 12 shows a comparison between two individuals belonging to different biotypes. The first FFO is a female fire biotype with a blood type O, while the second, AMA, is a male air biotype with an A blood type. According to the respective theories, the fire biotype is considered physically stronger than an air biotype (fire is considered as an athletic body type [mesomorph], while air is more an intellectual, smaller bone and muscle mass [ectomorph]).

To be crystal clear, an air biotype (similarly to a water biotype [endomorphs]) would never be able to contend productively in any kind of sports, given their low resistance and physical structural weakness (thin bone and muscle mass structure). On the contrary, a fire (athlete) and earth (strong and large body build like that of a "body builder") biotype are naturally shaped (as mesomorphs) to be able to compete in athletic (fire) and strength-related (earth) sports. Temperamental and psychological aspects of each biotype are also characteristic of their particular constitution: hormonal

p. 116/193

levels are constitutive of peculiar body shapes and forms. In this example, as an air biotype (cerebrotonic) the male is more concerned in intellectual activities, while a fire (or earth) biotype is more somatotonic, having complex traits associated with functional and anatomical predominance (more muscular prowess).

6 ABO Blood Type Diet

We shall avail ourselves of the therapeutic doctrine of the Hippocratic corpus in the definition or the possible remedies in kind which are to be prescribed for the healthy man to maintain or to improve his health as to patients suffering from a nosologically defined disease. The diet (in Greek, diaita), as a therapeutic instrument, includes the whole regimen (in Greek, diaitemata) of food. This is seen structured in gruel (a soup) and solids, drink (fluids), exercise, and baths.

The ABO-PLUS™ dietary suggestions concern both normal food (standard food items sold in the marketplace) and supplements (micronutrients like vitamins and minerals). These are the two columns that sustain the ABO-PLUS™ dietary intervention.

By experimentation many authors in the past 40 years have come up with a diet that is tailored to each individual's blood type. The most incredible thing about these BTDs is that they agree with each other in the types of foods that are to be eaten by each blood group individuals.

In the following pages, a diet suggestion is described for each blood type. This dietary pattern has been devised after many years of investigation and experimentation for both diseased and healthy people. Of course, this is just a general guide that can be even more customized (since we are all different and we might have issues with specific ingredients/ foods). We decided to mention only fresh, healthy, whole food, since we all know that, during cheat meal day, we might eat processed food, sugary chocolates, etc. Following a list of foods that might be beneficial based on your blood type.

6.1   A Diet for each Blood Type

An improved method of dieting for Blood Type Diet is presented hereafter based on each blood type. For each blood type, three diets are presented: these are divided into three steps. The first step is a relaxed diet where the major food types that should be consumed are indicated, and some less helpful foods are allowed. The second step is a stricter diet as more deleterious foods are removed. Finally, the last step is the strictest ABO blood type diet generally used only for severe symptoms.

All diets are further subdivided by their use on healthy and sick people, of course, the latter will need to have a stricter diet (preferring animal proteins [fish, eggs, meat] over carbohydrates). When sick people are considered, it is not to mean that they have a fever or other acute form of disease (although it is applicable to them too), but it is meant to identify those people who in one way or another have health problems.

No matter what blood type an individual has, it is important to:

1 Listen to each person's body signals;

2 Pay attention to each person's own food intolerances, sensitivities and/or allergies;

3 Pay attention to gluten and to animal milk and dairy products; it is better to reduce them or completely avoid them. The ABO lifestyle suggests avoiding foods containing gluten, lactose, or milk proteins;

4 Follow the correct food combinations and eat specific foods in the correct moment of the day (chrono diet).

5 Last but not least, always ask to your Medical Doctor for further details, since your MD knows you better.

The body always sends signals of health and disease that we must understand and heed. Bad signals are symptoms like fatigue, fever, pain, inflammation, headache, acne, bloating, nausea, etc.; while good signals are joy, energy, body flexibility, concentration, etc. Being able to follow the signs that the body sends to us is the first step to improving health.

The second step is not to blindly follow cliches and pre-ordained patterns. Even if a food is beneficial, or neutral, based on a specific blood type a person has (or indicated for most people), it does not mean that it is good for that person. If it is ascertained, based on the challenge-dechallenge-rechallenge (CDR) protocol, that an individual is intolerant or allergic to a specific food (or drink), that person MUST NOT EAT IT. It is appropriate to have a test to check potential foods intolerances since food intolerances can cause autoimmune diseases and other problems. For example, if an individual is intolerant to grass family, do not use sugar cane (oddly so, white sugar is better, anyway, than sugar cane – since white sugar comes from the beetroot family).

The third step would be to avoid eating foods that are known to be detrimental to an individual's health. Gluten is a protein contained in wheat and most grains (including Kamut, spelt, einkorn, emmer, barley, triticale, rye, oat, couscous, seitan). Gluten is like glue, and it sticks to intestine's walls, arteries, etc. There is no need for a person to be celiac to have problems with gluten, it is sufficient to be sensitive to it (unfortunately, even blood test, most of the time, cannot reveal this sensitivity) by causing minor and serious diseases (gut inflammation, Alzheimer, thyroid disorders, fibromyalgia, several autoimmune diseases, acid reflux, damage to gut flora, gas, ulcerative colitis, Crohn's, brain fog, dermatitis, etc.). Gluten free cereals are better, but they have to be eaten with moderation (if you are blood type O, B or AB, you should not eat corn): millet, rice, corn. Pseudo-grains are even better than gluten free cereals, although one should not exaggerate with their consumption: quinoa, amaranth, buckwheat (the last one only during the wintertime because it can warm up the body; but be careful with buckwheat if you have diabetes). Finally, dairy products (and milk proteins) can cause sore throat, inflammation, leaky gut syndrome, damage to gut flora, mucous, autoimmune diseases – especially when combined with gluten products consumption – etc., even if you have the natural enzyme lactase.

The fourth step is to try to avoid, when possible, a few food combinations. That means that it would be beneficial not to mix and match these categories of food during your meal (especially at dinner and if you have digestive issues). It is fine if on your cheat meal day you mix them if you do not have issues with that. Among these common potentially damaging combinations are:

i. Grains (both gluten free and with gluten) + Legumes (beans, pulses, e.g., lentils, broad beans, chickpeas, etc.);

ii. Grains (both gluten free and with gluten) + fruits (e.g., apples, apricots, chestnuts, cherries, etc.);

iii. Grains (both gluten free and with gluten) + sugars (white sugar, sugar cane, honey, agave, sweeteners, etc.);

iv. Grains (both gluten free and with gluten) + red meat (e.g., beef, calf, lamb, venison, duck, goat, etc.);

v. Grains (both gluten free and with gluten) + potatoes;

vi. Grains (both gluten free and with gluten) + squash/ pumpkin/ parsnip/ roots;

vii. Grains (both gluten free and with gluten) + chestnuts;

viii. Dairy products + chestnuts;

ix. Grains (both gluten free and with gluten) + dairy products;

x. Fruits + dairy products;

xi. Legumes/ beans/ pulses + dairy products;

xii. Meat + dairy products;

xiii. Grains (both gluten free and with gluten) + vinegar;

xiv. Grains (both gluten free and with gluten) + another grain;

xv. Rice and Millet never to be combined with tomato, lemon, wine, pumpkin;

xvi. Carrots are better during the day, preferably not with grains/ dairy products/ fruits;

xvii. No rice milk during pregnancy and lactation (it develops maltodextrin)

As already specified earlier, quinoa, amaranth and buckwheat are NOT considered GRAINS but pseudo-grains (pseudo-cereals) and can replace grains (always test that a person is able to digest them and is not intolerant):

1. They can be combined with fruit, dark chocolate, and sugar (e.g., cakes) but without exaggerating! This combination can be used at breakfast or as a treat;

2. Buckwheat is not good if you have thyroid issues or diabetes since it contains a lot of carbohydrates (hence, sugars);

3. Quinoa needs to be rinsed carefully to eliminate saponins. Do not eat quinoa if you are breastfeeding and if under 2 years of age. It might cause tummy pain because of the saponins;

4. Buckwheat can be eaten only during the cold season (autumn, winter) because it can warm you too much;

5. Amaranth is not suggested to blood type B;

6. They can be used with nuts (almonds, walnuts, hazelnuts, etc.), if you are not allergic to them.

The timing of the meal and the specific food items to be used is also important (chrono diet). Cereals (grains) and pseudo-cereals (and their relevant flours, pasta, etc.), and starch in general (sweet potatoes, beans, etc.) should be eaten only at breakfast and/or at lunch – better if combined with animal proteins (not red meat) and vegetables. This trick will allow the body to use carbohydrates during the day instead of storing them during the night. Similarly, legumes (pulses, soya, beans, etc.) might be preferably eaten only at breakfast and/or lunch – again, better if combined with animal proteins (poultry, fish, eggs) and vegetables. If someone wishes to lose weight, it is better to consume them no more than 3 times per week. Nuts can be combined pretty with everything if you can tolerate them.

Fruits should be eaten only at breakfast – better if combined with animal proteins or nuts (if tolerated). Do not exaggerate with fruit: fructose can cause inflammation. Roots (e.g., sweet potatoes, parsnip, pumpkin, swede, etc.) should be eaten only at breakfast and/ or lunch – better with animal proteins and vegetables. Vegetables three times per day. Other essential strategies are:

i. Animal proteins (meat, fish, and eggs) and vegetables can be eaten at breakfast, lunch, dinner, but please listen to your body, since we are all different;

ii. Drink hot water when you wake up, half an hour or one hour before your breakfast;

iii. Drink before meals and not too much during meals (unless it is a sip of water to swallow a big bite). Chew well. Drinking during meals fills up the stomach that cannot properly digest the food, especially animal proteins. The stomach has a capacity of 0,5 L if empty, and an average capacity of about 1 – 1.5 L if full. After a meal it will be expanded by 1 L to contain the bolus. If you force it to expand further, because of the intake of an excess of liquid during main meal, it will compress the abdomen and the chest creating heaviness, indigestion, and other problems. Drink if you are thirsty;

iv. Alcohol with moderation (better not to drink alcoholic drink if there are diseases and hepatitis);

v. Remember: sugary food is a treat. If you have diabetes, immune disease, flu, or any other kind of illness, please cut with sugar;

vi. Mushrooms: if you have issues with your liver (example: hepatitis) it would be better not to eat them, otherwise with moderation.

One final word of advice concerning diets in general is that one should carefully read the labels on the foods (especially ready meals and processed food, they might contain hidden bad ingredients). This is because often there are other substances that are more chemical and/or synthetic rather than natural added to the food item. Examples are:

i. Pork, monosodium glutamate (MSG), maltodextrin, gluten, lactose, dairy products, milk proteins, xylitol, maltitol, acesulfame K, aspartame, saccharine, added glucose and fructose, corn syrup, artificial sweeteners in general;

ii. Cut sugars and avoid brown sugar (if you are allergic to grass family, if you suffer of hay fever, then brown sugar and many grains/cereals with gluten are not good for you);

iii. When you read "sugar free" or "no added sugar", pay attention to the sweetener (the most acceptable are Stevia, Erythritol and Inulin);

iv. If you have issues with thyroid, please avoid or reduce the consumption of soya, seaweed, buckwheat, carob, chocolate, fruit, starches, honey, chestnuts, all kinds of potatoes, milk and dairy products, and sweets. Theoretically, quinoa and amaranth might be used after 6 months of accurate nutritional regime but moderately and only if you are under weight. It is better to eat legumes/ beans/ pulses than grains and pseudo-cereals (quinoa and amaranth). Eat pumpkin and squash, broccoli, cauliflower, cabbage and Brussels's sprouts with moderation, coffee with moderation. Chicory coffee might be a good alternative;

vii. If you have severe immune diseases, please avoid grains (with gluten and gluten free), and dairy products. Reduce drastically (even completely if you are in a serious condition) the consumption of carob, chocolate, fruit, sugar, fructose and sweets;

viii. Nowadays, supermarkets and wholefood shops sell pasta made with peas, chickpeas, mungo beans, etc. They can be used 2/3 times per week instead of standard pasta. You can also add nuts (if you do not have allergies);

ix. Be careful with hemp seeds if you have low blood pressure;

x. Instead of butter, you can use ghee, as it is lactose and casein free.

As always, once the general rules are set up, the most important thing is to listen to your body and its signals and test what is beneficial to you. Again, these are only general rules which should be adapted to your own personal needs. It is not necessary to follow them every day, or 100%. Just give it a try, without stressing yourself too much. If you see that you get improvements just applying these suggestions only at breakfast, for example, or at dinner, then stick to them.

It is a good practice to keep (especially the first month) a diary in which you write what you have eaten and drunk at breakfast/ lunch/ dinner/ snacks – to understand better what is good for your health and performance. Please, the first month do not have many things in the same plate. It is good to have one kind of animal protein, one kind of vegetable and (if it is not evening) one kind of beans, if you wish to have beans, OR allowed grains (if you wish them and if you can have it, but not at dinner), or other starches (pumpkin, sweet potato, etc.)

It is fundamental to contact your GP to ask for a blood test to identify your blood type if you do not have this information. This will allow you to customize the nutritional plan to your genetic makeup. This way the dietary pattern will work with your epigenetics and the new nutritional plan will be able to provide a better impact to your health. As always, listen to your body, to your reactions and, if you know to be sensitive or allergic to a food, do not eat it (I know it is obvious, but it is better to highlight it).

Ask always to your personal Medical Doctor for advice.

6.2 Blood Type A

6.2.1 General

Blood Type A people are more oriented towards poultry, fish, and eggs, together with vegetables, and some fruit. However, too many sugary products, too much fruit, too many grains/ cereals (even if gluten free) can create problems to your mood, your energy level, etc. It is also better to avoid dairy products (e.g., milk, cheese, cream, ice-cream, etc.). Do not mix meat and fish as this requires a lot of enzymes to be produced and dumped into the stomach by the liver and pancreas (it may cause indigestion).

It is healthier if you do not fry your food. Drink when you are thirsty.

Type A immune system is not very robust, and it usually takes more time to realize that a food is not well tolerated (unless the sensitivity is particularly high) and it takes more time to fully recover or to feel better.

It is healthier if you do not fry your food. Drink when you are thirsty.

A moderate exercise is fine (unless your GP/ Doctor suggests you not to). Practice sports that can help you to relax (e.g., yoga or Pilates) and try to rest when it is possible.

At least 30 minutes before having breakfast, get a cup (or two) of hot water with half squeezed lemon. You can also drink the hot water of the vegetables half an hour or 1 hour before your meal.

You can eat fresh vegetables as a snack together with some beans (beans only until lunch and never together with grains or roots). You can also eat sliced cooked poultry at breakfast, lunch, snack, or dinner (but dairy free, gluten free, potato starch free, corn starch/ flour free). Dried fruit (almond, prunes, natural almond butter) are good as snacks.

6.2.2 Healthy People

Meat

Neutral: capon, chicken, turkey, rooster, guinea-hen, ostrich.

Fish

Good: salmon, cod, sardines, mackerel, rainbow trout, carp, stone bass, perch.

Neutral: tuna, swordfish, trout, sea bass, smooth-hound, pike, white fish.

Milk and dairy product

(Better to avoid, otherwise it has to be a "treat", never together with cereals/ grains/ etc.)

Neutral: feta (from goat milk or sheep milk), goat cheese, mozzarella, goat ricotta, ricotta, goat yoghurt.

Soya

Good: soya milk, tofu (gluten free), soya yoghurt

Eggs

Good: from 4 to 6 eggs per week, preferably not fried.

Cereals and grains

(and relevant flour)

p. 127/193

Good: amaranth, buckwheat (only in autumn/ winter), kasha (toasted buckwheat).

Neutral: quinoa. Rice, corn, tapioca, and millet to be used much less than the previous pseudo cereals.

Oils and Fats

Good: extra-virgin olive oil, grape seed oil, linseed oil, pumpkin seed oil, rice oil.

Neutral: sesame oil, sunflower oil, hempseed oil.

Seeds

(Walnuts and chestnuts only during autumn and winter)

Good: peanuts, peanut butter, walnuts, and pumpkin seeds.

Neutral: chestnuts (better not to eat them with cereals – even gluten free grains – and dairy products), pine nuts, almonds, macadamia nuts, pecan, hemp seeds, sesame seeds, sunflower seeds and butter, almond butter, walnut butter, hazelnut butter, tahini.

Use these kinds of butter with moderation.

Legumes/ beans/ pulses

You can use also beans flours (you can prepare it or use cooked beans to be mixed with eggs and other ingredient to bake bread or cake for daytime meals) – together with poultry, eggs, or fish. Nowadays, you can also find legumes pasta (for personal experience, it is better not to have them more than 2/3 times per week – however, you should test on yourself).

Good: adzuki (red soya), black eyed beans, black beans, lentils, red lentils, yellow and green soya.

Neutral: cannellini beans, green beans (you can eat these also at dinner), peas (you can eat these also at dinner), broad beans, mange tout, lupin bean.

Vegetables

(at least three times per day)

p. 128/193

Good: chards, broccoli, artichokes, chicory, carrots, onion, parsnip, alfalfa sprouts, soya sprouts, parsley (fresh, not cooked), leak, spinach, turnip, dandelion, pumpkin, beet tops, squash, savoy cabbage, Jerusalem's artichoke, endive.

Neutral: seaweed, asparagus, beetroot, cauliflower, Brussels' sprouts, cucumber, cabbage, daikon, fennel, porcini, green olives, red radicchio, radish, rocket, shallot, celery, black/ white truffle, courgette.

Reminder:

- Garlic only if you can digest it;
- Artichoke, lettuce, spinach: to be avoided if without gallbladder;
- Onion only if you can digest it.

Fruit

(moderately, only at breakfast and with animal proteins or nuts)

Good: figs (fresh and dry), plums, prunes (check the label: no added sugar), apricot, pineapple, cherry, grapefruit, sultana, lemons, blackberry.

Neutral: watermelon, avocado, Sharon fruit/ persimmon, carob, dates, kiwi, raspberry, lemon (on fish), pomegranate, apple, blueberry, papaya, prickly pear, peach, pear, grapefruit, grape, gooseberry, blackcurrant, redcurrant, elder.

Jam: alone, as a snack, or with animal proteins. Jam never together with cereals/ roots/ flours.

Juices

(same rules as per fruit) with moderation, only during summer and no added sugar in them.

Good: apricot, pineapple, carrot, lemon, blueberry, grapefruit, cherry, plum.

Neutral: savoy cabbage, grape, pear, apple.

p. 129/193

Spices

Good: tamari sauce (gluten free), soya miso (gluten free), mustard (without vinegar), ginger.

Neutral: bay laurel, aniseed, basil, bergamot, cinnamon, coriander, cumin, turmeric, curry, fennel seeds, rosemary, sage, salt, thyme, chives, brewer's yeast, nutmeg, saffron, mint.

Sweets

(moderately, sugar/ sweetener free, gluten free, lactose free, milk free)

Good: molasses.

Neutral: carob, carob powder, rice drink, soya drink, almond drink, maple syrup, agave syrup, white sugar, dark chocolate, dark hazelnut chocolate, stevia, inulin.

Honey far from meals and in herbal teas or with animal proteins

Sauce/ pesto/ chutney/ paste

(you can prepare the sauce you like)

Neutral: artichoke paste, green olive paste, basil pesto (dairy and gluten free), mayo (without vinegar), jam/ marmalade with allowed fruit, parsley and soya sauce, mustard without vinegar.

Drinks

(NO BLACK TEA)

Good: still water (room temperature), chicory coffee, green tea, bancha tea, red wine (with moderation, at lunch, it can be used to cook instead of the oil), vegetable water (at least half an hour before a meal), dandelion, rosehip, propolis, ginger.

Neutral: coffee (moderately), ginseng, fennel tea, chamomile, karkadè, white wine (moderately and only at lunch, it can be used to cook instead of the oil).

Herbs

Good: alfalfa sprouts, Aloe vera, Roman chamomile, chamomile, ginger, dandelion, rosehip, ginger, St. John's wort, propolis, valerian.

Neutral: birch, calendula, sage (not to be used if you are pregnant or breastfeeding, daytime only), hawthorn, linden, fennel seeds, strawberry, raspberry, mulberry, peppermint, parsley, liquorice root (if blood pressure is not high), verbena.

6.2.3 People with severe symptoms

Meat

Neutral: capon, chicken, turkey, rooster, guinea-hen, ostrich.

Fish

Good: salmon, cod, sardines, mackerel, rainbow trout, carp, stone bass, perch.

Neutral: tuna, swordfish, trout, sea bass, smooth-hound, pike, white fish.

Soya

(Not to be used if taking medicines for thyroid issues) – no added sugar/ sweeteners.

Good: soya milk, tofu (gluten free), soya yoghurt

Eggs

Good: from 4 to 6 eggs per week, not fried (no butter with them).

Cereals and grains

(and relevant flour)

Good: amaranth, buckwheat (only in autumn/ winter), kasha (toasted buckwheat).

Neutral: quinoa.

Oils and Fats

p. 131/193

Good: extra-virgin olive oil, grape seed oil, linseed oil, pumpkin seed oil, rice oil.

Neutral: sesame oil, sunflower oil, hempseed oil.

Seeds

(walnuts and chestnuts only during autumn and winter)

Good: peanuts, peanut butter, walnuts, pumpkin seeds.

Neutral: pine nuts, almonds, macadamia nuts, pecan, chestnuts, hemp seeds, sesame seeds, sunflower seeds and butter, almond butter, walnut butter, hazelnut butter, tahini.

All these kinds of butter must be used with moderation.

Legumes/ beans/ pulses

You can use also beans flours (you can prepare it or use cooked beans to be mixed with eggs and other ingredient to bake bread or cake for daytime meals) – together with poultry, eggs, or fish. You can buy legumes pasta.

Good: adzuki (red soya), black eyed beans, black beans, lentils, red lentils, yellow and green soya.

Neutral: cannellini beans, green beans (you can eat these also at dinner), peas (you can eat these also at dinner), broad beans, mange tout, lupin bean.

Vegetables

(at least three times per day)

Good: chards, broccoli, artichokes, chicory, carrots, onion, parsnip, alfalfa sprouts, soya sprouts, parsley (fresh, not cooked), leak, spinach, turnip, dandelion, pumpkin, beet tops, squash, savoy cabbage, Jerusalem's artichoke, endive.

Neutral: seaweed, asparagus, beetroot, cauliflower, Brussels' sprouts, cucumber, cabbage, daikon, fennel, porcini, green olives, red radicchio, radish, rocket, shallot, celery, black/ white truffle, courgette.

Reminder:

- Garlic only if you can digest it;
- Artichoke, lettuce, spinach: to be avoided if without gallbladder;
- Onion only if you can digest it.

Spices

Good: tamari sauce (gluten free), soya miso (gluten free), mustard (without vinegar), ginger.

Neutral: bay laurel, aniseed, basil, bergamot, cinnamon, coriander, cumin, turmeric, curry, fennel seeds, rosemary, sage, salt, thyme, chives, brewer's yeast, nutmeg, saffron, mint.

Sauce/ pesto/ chutney/ paste

(you can prepare the sauce you like)

Neutral: artichoke paste, green olive paste, basil pesto (dairy and gluten free), mayo (without vinegar), jam/ marmalade with allowed fruit, parsley and soya sauce, mustard without vinegar.

Drinks

(NO BLACK TEA)

Good: still water (room temperature), chicory coffee, green tea, bancha tea, red wine (with moderation, at lunch, it can be used to cook instead of the oil), vegetable water (at least half an hour before a meal), dandelion, rosehip, propolis, ginger.

Neutral: coffee (moderately), ginseng, fennel tea, chamomile, karkadè, white wine (moderately and only at lunch, it can be used to cook instead of the oil).

Herbs

Good: alfalfa sprouts, Aloe vera, Roman chamomile, chamomile, ginger, dandelion, rosehip, ginger, St. John's wort, propolis, valerian.

Neutral: birch, calendula, sage (not to be used if you are pregnant or breastfeeding, daytime only), hawthorn, linden, fennel seeds, strawberry, raspberry, mulberry, peppermint, parsley, liquorice root (if blood pressure is not high), verbena.

6.3   Blood Type B

6.3.1 General

Blood Type B has generally a good immune system, but autoimmune diseases and blood issues can be developed. Blood Type B's motto is: "fewer foods per meal". Avoid corn, tomato, gluten, chicken and pork: they can be dangerous for you. You get stressed easily but you are able to manage it once good food is introduced. Sport is good but it is better if it does not require too much effort. Do not mix meat and fish as this requires a lot of enzymes to be produced and dumped into the stomach by the liver and pancreas (it may cause indigestion).

It is healthier if you do not fry your food. Drink when you are thirsty.

It is important for you to exercise (unless your GP/ Doctor suggests you not to). Sport helps you to reduce stress and diseases. A moderate exercise is fine (unless your GP/ Doctor suggests you not to). Practice sports and something that can help you to relax (e.g., yoga or Pilates) and try to rest when it is possible.

Similarly, to other blood types, at least 30 minutes before having breakfast, get a cup (or two) of hot water with half squeezed lemon. You can also drink the hot water of the vegetables half an hour or 1 hour before your meal.

You can eat fresh vegetables as a snack together with some beans (beans only until lunch and never together with cereals or roots). You can also eat sliced cooked poultry at breakfast, lunch, snack, or dinner (but dairy free, gluten free, potato starch free, corn starch/ flour free). Dried fruit (almond, prunes) are good as snacks.

6.3.2 Healthy People

Meat

Good: lamb, goat, roe deer, venison, rabbit, mutton, deer

Neutral: beef or horse bresaola (dairy free, sugar free, gluten free – read the labels), horse, liver (from beef), beef, calf, turkey, pheasant, ostrich.

Fish

Good: caviar, stone bass, Halibut, pike, cod, hake, salmon, sardines, mackerel, sole, sturgeon.

Neutral: rainbow trout, trout, swordfish, herring, tuna, gilthead bream (orate), squid (calamari), scallop, smooth-hound, perch, cuttlefish/ squid, goatfish, white fish.

Milk and dairy product

(These products are tolerated best by this blood type but never together with cereals/ grains/ etc.)

You should AVOID MILK AND DAIRY PRODUCTS: ovarian/ breast/ uterus/ prostate cancer, prostate issues, kidney stones, gallstones. In case of colitis the quantity must be reduced or avoided at all. It is better to use goat dairy products than cow dairy products. No whipped cream, no cream, no mascarpone, no hard cheese, no fatty cheese (gorgonzola, etc.).

Good: feta (from goat or sheep), milk flakes, goat cheese, fresh light cheese, kefir, goat skimmed milk, skimmed milk, mozzarella, light ricotta, yogurt.

Neutral: Brie, butter, camembert, cheddar, Edam, Emmenthal, ice-cream, whole goat's milk, whole cow's milk, Parmesan (Parmigiano), Provolone.

Soya

Good: soya milk, tofu (gluten free), soya yoghurt

Eggs

Good: from 4 to 6 eggs per week, better if not fried (butter is allowed).

Cereals and grains

(and relevant flour)

Good: millet, quinoa, rice (puffed, black, red, whole/ brown, wild).

Neutral: gluten free oat, potato starch, Muesli, basmati rice, white rice.

Rice and Millet not to be used with lemon and/ or wine.

Oils and Fats

Good: grape seed oil, rice oil.

Neutral: butter, cod liver oil, linseed oil, extra-virgin olive oil, hempseed oil.

Seeds

(walnuts and chestnuts only during autumn and winter)

Neutral: chestnuts, almonds, Brazil nuts, pecan nuts, walnuts, macadamia nuts, hemp seeds, almond butter, and walnut butter.

All these kinds of butter to be used with moderation.

Chestnuts: do not combine them with cereals/ grains, dairy products. To be avoided during the summertime.

Legumes/ beans/ pulses

You can use also beans flours (you can prepare it or use cooked beans to be mixed with eggs and other ingredient to bake bread or cake for daytime meals) – together with poultry, eggs, or fish.

Good: butter beans, Lima beans.

Neutral: kidney beans, cannellini beans, red beans, green beans (you can eat these also at dinner), peas (you can eat these also at dinner), broad beans, yellow and green soya, mange tout.

Vegetables

(at least three times per day)

Good: beetroot, broccoli, cauliflower, Brussels sprouts, onion, parsnip, sweet potatoes, cabbage, leak, spinach, savoy cabbage, peppers, parsley, carrots.

Neutral: alfa-alfa sprouts, seaweed, asparagus, dill, kohlrabi, chicory, onion, cucumber, chervil, daikon, fennel, porcini mushrooms, soya sprouts, endive, chestnut mushroom, lettuce (summer), leek, celery, radish, horseradish, spinach, courgette/zucchini, ginger, chard, potatoes, dandelion, turnip.

Reminder:

- Garlic only if you can digest it;
- Artichoke, lettuce, spinach: to be avoided if without gallbladder;
- Onion only if you can digest it.

Fruit

(moderately, only at breakfast and with animal proteins or nuts)

Good: pineapple, banana, red berry, Papaya, plums, prunes (check the label: no added sugar), grape.

Neutral: apricot, watermelon, orange, tangerine, cherry, figs, dates, kiwi, raspberry, lemon, mango, apple, blueberry, melon, peach, pear, grapefruit, grape, blackcurrant, sultana, elder.

Jam: alone, as a snack, or with animal proteins (e.g.: omelettes). Jam never together with cereals/ roots/ flours/ dairy products.

Juices

(same rules as per fruit) with moderation, only during summer

Good: pineapple, cabbage, Papaya, grape, blueberry.

Neutral: apricot, orange, carrot, grapefruit, plum, cherry, apple.

Spices

Good: ginger, horseradish, curry, cayenne pepper.

Neutral: bay laurel, aniseed, basil, bergamot, cappers, carob, cardamom, chervil, coriander, cumin, fennel seeds, pepper, rosemary, sage, salt, tarragon, mustard, marjoram, gluten free soya sauce, thyme, chives, cloves, miso, saffron, black pepper, dill, mint, nutmeg, peppermint, vanilla.

• Paprika, black pepper, chili pepper, salt to be used with moderation.

Sweets

(moderately, sugar/ sweetener free, gluten free, lactose free, milk free)

Neutral: chocolate (without hazelnuts). rice drink, millet drink, carob, carob powder, molasses, almond drink, maple syrup, white sugar, stevia, inulin.

Honey far from meals and in herbal teas or with animal proteins

Sauce/ pesto/ chutney/ paste

(you can prepare the sauce you like)

Neutral: mayonnaise (without corn starch), basil pesto (dairy and gluten free if possible), jam/ marmalade with allowed fruit, mustard, parsley, sweet and sour vegetables.

Drinks

(NO BLACK TEA)

Good: still water (room temperature), chicory coffee, green tea.

Neutral: coffee (with moderation), rice beer and millet beer (gluten free, barley free, wheat free), ginseng (with moderation), karkadè, red wine and white wine (moderately and only at lunch, it can be used to cook instead of the oil).

p. 138/193

Herbs

Good: Roman chamomile, Ginseng, liquorice root (if blood pressure is not high), peppermint, passionflower, propolis, rosehip, sage, ginger

Neutral: burdock, hawthorn, chamomile, calendula, mint, Echinacea, dandelion, hypericum, valerian, fennel seed, thyme, elder.

6.3.3 People with severe symptoms

Meat

Good: lamb, goat, roe deer, venison, rabbit, mutton, deer

Neutral: beef or horse bresaola (dairy free, sugar free, gluten free – read the labels), horse, liver (from beef), beef, calf, turkey, pheasant, ostrich.

Fish

Good: caviar, stone bass, Halibut, pike, cod, hake, salmon, sardines, mackerel, sole, sturgeon.

Neutral: rainbow trout, trout, swordfish, herring, tuna, gilthead bream (orate), squid (calamari), scallop, smooth-hound, perch, cuttlefish/ squid, goatfish, white fish.

Soya

Good: soya milk, tofu (gluten free), soya yoghurt

Eggs

Good: from 4 to 6 eggs per week, not fried (butter is allowed).

Oils and Fats

Good: grape seed oil, rice oil.

Neutral: butter, cod liver oil, linseed oil, extra-virgin olive oil, hempseed oil.

Seeds

(walnuts and chestnuts only during autumn and winter)

Neutral: chestnuts, almonds, Brazil nuts, pecan nuts, walnuts, macadamia nuts, hemp seeds, almond butter, and walnut butter.

All these kinds of butter have to be used with moderation.

Chestnuts: do not combine them with cereals/ grains, dairy products. To be avoided during the summertime.

Legumes/ beans/ pulses

You can use also beans flours (you can prepare it or use cooked beans to be mixed with eggs and other ingredient to bake bread or cake for daytime meals) – together with poultry, eggs, or fish.

Good: butter beans, Lima beans.

Neutral: kidney beans, cannellini beans, red beans, green beans (you can eat these also at dinner), peas (you can eat these also at dinner), broad beans, yellow and green soya, mange tout.

Vegetables

(at least three times per day)

Good: beetroot, broccoli, cauliflower, Brussels sprouts, onion, parsnip, sweet potatoes, cabbage, leak, spinach, savoy cabbage, peppers, parsley, carrots.

Neutral: alfa-alfa sprouts, seaweed, asparagus, dill, kohlrabi, chicory, onion, cucumber, chervil, daikon, fennel, porcini mushrooms, soya sprouts, endive, chestnut mushroom, lettuce (summer), leek, celery, radish, horseradish, spinach, courgette/ zucchini, ginger, chard, potatoes, dandelion, turnip.

Reminder:

- Garlic only if you can digest it;
- Artichoke, lettuce, spinach: to be avoided if without gallbladder;
- Onion only if you can digest it.

Spices

Good: ginger, horseradish, curry, cayenne pepper.

Neutral: bay laurel, aniseed, basil, bergamot, cappers, carob, cardamom, chervil, coriander, cumin, fennel seeds, pepper, rosemary, sage, salt, tarragon, mustard, marjoram, gluten free soya sauce, thyme, chives, cloves, miso, saffron, black pepper, dill, mint, nutmeg, peppermint, vanilla.

• Paprika, black pepper, chili pepper, salt to be used with moderation.

Sweets

(moderately, sugar/ sweetener free, gluten free, lactose free, milk free)

Neutral: chocolate (without hazelnuts), rice drink, millet drink, carob, carob powder, molasses, almond drink, maple syrup, white sugar, stevia, inulin.

Honey far from meals and in herbal teas or with animal proteins

Sauce/ pesto/ chutney/ paste

(you can prepare the sauce you like)

Neutral: mayonnaise (without corn starch), basil pesto (dairy and gluten free if possible), jam/ marmalade with allowed fruit, mustard, parsley, sweet and sour vegetables.

Drinks

(NO BLACK TEA)

Good: still water (room temperature), chicory coffee, green tea.

Neutral: coffee (with moderation), ginseng (with moderation).

Herbs

Good: Roman chamomile, Ginseng, liquorice root (if blood pressure is not high), peppermint, passionflower, propolis, rosehip, sage, ginger

Neutral: burdock, hawthorn, chamomile, calendula, mint, Echinacea, dandelion, hypericum, valerian, fennel seed, thyme, elder.

6.4   Blood Type O

6.4.1 General

Blood Type O is carnivore. Red meat, poultry, fish, and eggs, together with vegetables, are the best food for you. Too many sugary products, too much fruit, too many cereals (even if gluten free) can create problems to your mood, your energy level, your stomach, etc. It is better to avoid dairy products (e.g., milk, cheese, cream, ice-cream, etc.). Do not mix meat and fish as this requires a lot of enzymes to be produced and dumped into the stomach by the liver and pancreas (it may cause indigestion).

It is healthier if you do not fry your food. Drink when you are thirsty.

It is easy for you to react to something you do not tolerate but, at the same time, you can recover/ feel better quicker if you eat what is good for you. It is healthier if you do not fry your food. Drink when you are thirsty.

A moderate exercise is fine (unless your GP/ Doctor suggests you not to). Practice sports and something can help you to relax (e.g., yoga or Pilates) and try to rest when it is possible.

At least 30 minutes before having breakfast, get a cup (or two) of hot water. You can also drink the hot water of the vegetables half an hour or 1 hour before your meal.

You can eat fresh vegetables as a snack together with some beans (beans only until lunch and never together with cereals or roots). You can also eat sliced cooked poultry at breakfast, lunch, snack, or dinner (but dairy free, gluten free, potato starch free, corn starch/ flour free). Dried fruit (almond, prunes) are good as snacks.

p. 142/193

6.4.2 Healthy People

Meat

Good: lamb, bresaola (dairy free, sugar free, gluten free – read the labels), goat, beef, venison, horse, calf, mutton, roe deer.

Neutral: duck, rabbit, hare, capon, chicken, turkey, rooster, pheasant, ostrich.

Fish

Good: cod, sardines, mackerel, rainbow trout, swordfish, herring, hake, sole, pike, sturgeon.

Neutral: tuna, salmon, trout, anchovy, carp, gilthead bream (orate), sea bass, oyster, lobster, clams, squid, crab, shrimp, prawn, goatfish, white fish.

Milk and dairy product

(Better to avoid, otherwise it has to be a "treat", never together with cereals/ grains/ etc.)

Neutral: feta (from goat milk or sheep milk), goat cheese, mozzarella.

Soya

Good: soya milk, tofu (gluten free), soya yoghurt

Eggs

Good: from 2 to 7 eggs per week, not fried (no butter with them).

Cereals and grains

(and relevant flour)

Neutral: amaranth, buckwheat (only in autumn/ winter), quinoa. Rice, tapioca, and millet to be used much less than the previous pseudo cereals.

Oils and Fats

Good: grape seed oil, linseed oil, pumpkin seed oil.

Neutral: butter (only in winter but without exaggerating), sesame oil, extra-virgin olive oil, soya oil, sunflower oil, hempseed oil.

Seeds

(walnuts and chestnuts only during autumn and winter)

Good: walnuts, pumpkin seeds.

Neutral: chestnuts (not to eat with cereals – even gluten free grains – and dairy products), almonds, macadamia nuts, pecan, hemp seeds, sesame seeds, sunflower seeds, almond butter, walnut butter, hazelnut butter, tahini.

All these kinds of butter have to be used with moderation.

Legumes/ beans/ pulses

You can use also beans flours (you can prepare it or use cooked beans to be mixed with eggs and other ingredient to bake bread or cake for daytime meals) – together with poultry, eggs, or fish.

Good: adzuki (red soya), black eyed beans.

Neutral: chickpea, cannellini beans, black and red beans, green beans (you can eat these also at dinner), peas (you can eat these also at dinner), broad beans, soya, mange tout, lupin bean.

Vegetables

(at least three times per day)

Good: seaweed, chards, broccoli, artichokes, chicory, onion, parsnip, turnip, sweet potatoes, savoy cabbage, leak, spinach, dandelion, pumpkin, beet tops, squash.

Neutral: asparagus, beetroot, carrots, cucumber, cabbage, daikon, fennel, porcini, soya sprouts, green olives, endive, lettuce (summer), radish, rocket, shallot, celery, black/ white truffle, Jerusalem's artichoke, ginger, courgette, pepper, tomato.

Reminder:

- Garlic only if you can digest it;

- Artichoke, lettuce, spinach: to be avoided if without gallbladder;
- Onion only if you can digest it.

Fruit

(moderately, only at breakfast and with animal proteins or nuts)

Good: figs (fresh and dry), plums, prunes (check the label: no added sugar)

Neutral: apricot, pineapple, watermelon, banana, Sharon fruit/ persimmon, cherry, dates, kiwi, raspberry, lemon (on fish), mango, pomegranate, apple, blueberry, papaya, prickly pear, peach, pear, grapefruit, grape, blackcurrant, sultana, elder.

Jam: alone, as a snack, or with animal proteins. Jam never together with cereals/ roots/ flours.

Juices

(same rules as per fruit) with moderation, only during summer

Good: pineapple, cherry, plum.

Neutral: blueberry, grape, carrot, grapefruit.

Spices

Good: turmeric, curry, cayenne pepper.

Neutral: bay laurel, aniseed, basil, bergamot, coriander, cumin, fennel seeds, pepper, rosemary, sage, salt, mustard without vinegar, gluten free soya sauce, thyme, chives, brewer's yeast, cloves, miso, saffron, black pepper, dill, mint.

- Paprika, black pepper, chili pepper to be used with moderation

Sweets

(moderately, sugar/ sweetener free, gluten free, lactose free, milk free)

Good: carob, carob powder.

Neutral: rice drink, soya drink, molasses, almond drink, maple syrup, sugar, dark chocolate, dark hazelnut chocolate, stevia, inulin.

Honey far from meals and in herbal teas or with animal proteins

Sauce/ pesto/ chutney/ paste

(you can prepare the sauce you like)

Neutral: artichoke paste, green olive paste, tomato sauce, basil pesto (dairy and gluten free), mayo (without vinegar), jam/ marmalade with allowed fruit.

Drinks

(NO COFFEE OR BLACK TEA)

Good: Roman chamomile, chamomile, peppermint, linden, ginger, dandelion, rosehip, mulberry, passionflower, propolis.

Neutral: chamomile, karkadè, green tea (exception and very light), red wine and white wine (moderately and only at lunch, it can be used to cook instead of the oil), rice beer (gluten free, barley free, wheat free).

Herbs

Good: Roman chamomile, chamomile, peppermint, linden, ginger, dandelion, rosehip, mulberry, passionflower, propolis.

Neutral: hawthorn, ginseng, liquorice root (if blood pressure is not high), parsley (not cooked), calendula, sage, fennel seed, thyme.

6.4.3 People with diseases

Meat

Good: lamb, bresaola (dairy free, sugar free, gluten free – read the labels), goat, beef, venison, horse, calf, mutton, roe deer.

Neutral: duck, rabbit, hare, capon, chicken, turkey, rooster, pheasant, ostrich.

p. 146/193

Fish

Good: cod, sardines, mackerel, rainbow trout, swordfish, herring, hake, sole, pike, sturgeon.

Neutral: tuna, salmon, trout, anchovy, carp, gilthead bream (orate), sea bass, oyster, lobster, clams, squid, crab, shrimp, prawn, goatfish, white fish.

Soya

Neutral: soya milk, tofu (gluten free), soya yoghurt

Eggs

Good: from 2 to 7 eggs per week, not fried (no butter with them).

Oils and Fats

Good: grape seed oil, linseed oil, pumpkin seed oil.

Neutral: butter (only in winter but without exaggerating), sesame oil, extra-virgin olive oil, soya oil, sunflower oil, hempseed oil.

Seeds

(walnuts and chestnuts only during autumn and winter)

Good: walnuts, pumpkin seeds.

Neutral: chestnuts (not to eat with cereals – even gluten free grains – and dairy products), almonds, macadamia nuts, pecan, hemp seeds, sesame seeds, sunflower seeds, almond butter, walnut butter, hazelnut butter, tahini.

All these kinds of butter have to be used with moderation.

Legumes/ beans/ pulses

You can use also beans flours (you can prepare it or use cooked beans to be mixed with eggs and other ingredient to bake bread or cake for daytime meals) – together with poultry, eggs, or fish.

Good: adzuki (red soya), black eyed beans.

Neutral: chickpea, cannellini beans, black and red beans, green beans (you can eat these also at dinner), peas (you can eat these also at dinner), broad beans, soya, mange tout, lupin bean.

Vegetables

(at least three times per day)

Good: seaweed, chards, broccoli, artichokes, chicory, onion, parsnip, turnip, sweet potatoes, savoy cabbage, leak, spinach, dandelion, pumpkin, beet tops, squash.

Neutral: asparagus, beetroot, carrots, cucumber, cabbage, daikon, fennel, porcini, soya sprouts, green olives, endive, lettuce (summer), radish, rocket, shallot, celery, black/ white truffle, Jerusalem's artichoke, ginger, courgette, pepper, tomato.

Reminder:

- Garlic only if you can digest it;
- Artichoke, lettuce, spinach: to be avoided if without gallbladder;
- Onion only if you can digest it.

Spices

Good: turmeric, curry, cayenne pepper.

Neutral: bay laurel, aniseed, basil, bergamot, coriander, cumin, fennel seeds, pepper, rosemary, sage, salt, mustard without vinegar, gluten free soya sauce, thyme, chives, brewer's yeast, cloves, miso, saffron, black pepper, dill, mint.

- Paprika, black pepper, chili pepper to be used with moderation

Sweets

(moderately, sugar/ sweetener free, gluten free, lactose free, milk free)

Good: carob, carob powder.

Neutral: stevia, inulin.

p. 148/193

Honey far from meals and in herbal teas or with animal proteins

Sauce/ pesto/ chutney/ paste

(you can prepare the sauce you like)

Neutral: artichoke paste, green olive paste, tomato sauce, basil pesto (dairy and gluten free), mayo (without vinegar), jam/ marmalade with allowed fruit.

Drinks

(NO COFFEE OR BLACK TEA)

Good: Roman chamomile, chamomile, peppermint, linden, ginger, dandelion, rosehip, mulberry, passionflower, propolis.

Neutral: chamomile, karkadè, green tea (exception and very light), red wine and white wine (moderately and only at lunch, it can be used to cook instead of the oil), rice beer (gluten free, barley free, wheat free).

Herbs

Good: Roman chamomile, chamomile, peppermint, linden, ginger, dandelion, rosehip, mulberry, passionflower, propolis.

Neutral: hawthorn, ginseng, liquorice root (if blood pressure is not high), parsley (not cooked), calendula, sage, fennel seed, thyme.

6.5   Blood Type AB

6.5.1 General

Blood Type AB has generally a weak immune system: it is open to virus and bacteria. Both negative reactions and recovery might take a long time. Because of this, AB type has to be accurate with diseases related to food, since an adverse reaction might happen after few days. A balanced life (food, relaxation, and lifestyle) can help AB to build the immune system. Sport and relaxation might to be alternated in AB type. It is important for you to exercise (unless your GP/ Doctor suggests you not to), but not performing strenuous sports.

Avoid corn, gluten, chickpeas, chicken, and pork: they can be dangerous for you. Do not mix meat and fish as this requires a lot of enzymes to be produced and dumped into the stomach by the liver and pancreas (it may cause indigestion).

It is healthier if you do not fry your food. Drink when you are thirsty.

A moderate exercise is fine (unless your GP/ Doctor suggests you not to). Practice sports and something that can help you to relax (e.g., yoga or Pilates) and try to rest when it is possible.

At least 30 minutes before having breakfast, get a cup (or two) of hot water with half squeezed lemon. You can also drink the hot water of the vegetables half an hour or 1 hour before your meal.

You can eat fresh vegetables as a snack together with some beans (beans only until lunch and never together with cereals or roots). You can also eat sliced cooked poultry at breakfast, lunch, snack, or dinner (but dairy free, gluten free, potato starch free, corn starch/ flour free). Dried fruit (almond, prunes) are good as snacks.

6.5.2 Healthy People

Meat

Good: lamb, goat, rabbit, venison, rabbit, mutton.

Neutral: pheasant, turkey, liver (from beef or turkey), ostrich.

Fish

Good: stone bass, pike, snails (Helix Pomatia), cod, hake, salmon, sardines, mackerel, tuna, sturgeon.

Neutral: herring, squid, caviar, carp, scallop, mussel, gilthead bream (orate), smooth-hound, perch, catfish, swordfish, cuttlefish/ squid, sole, rainbow trout, trout, goatfish, white fish.

p. 150/193

Milk and dairy product

(These products are somewhat tolerated by this blood type but never together with cereals/ grains/ etc.)

You should AVOID MILK AND DAIRY PRODUCTS: ovarian/ breast/ uterus/ prostate cancer, prostate issues, kidney stones, gallstones. In case of colitis the quantity has to be reduced or avoided at all. It is better to use goat dairy products than cow dairy products. No whipped cream, no cream, no mascarpone, no hard cheese, no fatty cheese (gorgonzola, etc.).

Good: feta (from goat or sheep), goat cheese, Mozzarella, light ricotta, goat yogurt.

Neutral: crescenza cheese, Edam, Emmenthal, skimmed goat milk (and flakes), skimmed cow milk (moderately), light yogurt (moderately).

Soya

Neutral: soya milk, tofu (gluten free), soya yoghurt

Eggs

Good: from 3 to 7 eggs per week, not fried (no butter with them).

Cereals and grains

(and relevant flour)

Good: millet, rice (puffed, black, basmati, red, whole/ brown, wild).

Neutral: amaranth, quinoa, gluten free oat, potato starch.

Rice and Millet not to be used with lemon and/ or wine.

Oils and Fats

Good: extra virgin olive oil, grape seed oil, rice oil.

Neutral: cod liver oil, linseed oil, hempseed oil.

Seeds

(walnuts and chestnuts only during autumn and winter)

Good: peanut, peanut butter, chestnuts, walnuts.

Neutral: almonds, Brazil nuts, pistachio, pine nuts, pecan nuts, macadamia nuts, hemp seeds, almond butter (to be used with moderation).

Chestnuts: do not combine them with cereals/ grains, dairy products. To be avoided during the summertime

Legumes/ beans/ pulses

You can use also beans flours (you can prepare it or use cooked beans to be mixed with eggs and other ingredient to bake bread or cake for daytime meals) – together with poultry, eggs, or fish.

Good: kidney beans, red beans, green lentils.

Neutral: cannellini beans, lentils and red lentils, peas, and green beans (you can eat these also at dinner), broad beans, yellow and green soya, mange tout, lupin beans.

Vegetables

(at least three times per day)

Good: alfa-alfa sprouts, beetroot, chard and Swiss chard, broccoli, cauliflower, cucumber, aubergine, parsnip, parsnip, sweet potatoes, celery, dandelion, parsley.

Neutral: seaweed, asparagus, carrot, Brussels sprouts, savoy cabbage, cabbage, chicory, chervil, daikon, fennel, watercress, cumin, porcini mushrooms, Bamboo sprouts, soya sprouts, endive, chestnut mushroom, green olives, lettuce (summer), leek, onion, radish, horseradish, spinach, courgette/ zucchini, ginger, truffle, pumpkin, potatoes.

Reminder:

- Garlic only if you can digest it;
- Artichoke, lettuce, spinach: to be avoided if without gallbladder;

p. 152/193

- Onion only if you can digest it.

Fruit

(moderately, only at breakfast and with animal proteins or nuts)

Good: pineapple, cherry, plums, grape, figs (fresh and dried), kiwi, lemon, grapefruit, gooseberry.

Neutral: apricot, watermelon, carob, dates, strawberry, tangerine (moderately), raspberry, apple, blueberry, melon, peach, pear, blackcurrant, prunes (check the label: no added sugar), raisin, Papaya, elder.

Jam: alone, as a snack, or with animal proteins (e.g.: omelettes). Jam never together with cereals/ roots/ flours/ dairy products.

Juices

(same rules as per fruit) with moderation, only during summer

Good: carrot, cabbage, cherry, Papaya, grape.

Neutral: water and lemon, apricot, pineapple, grapefruit, plum, apple.

Spices

Good: garlic, ginger, curry, horseradish.

Neutral: bay laurel, dill, bergamot, carob, basil, cinnamon, carob, cardamom, chervil, coriander, turmeric, cumin, fennel seeds, rosemary, sage, salt, tarragon, marjoram, gluten free soya sauce, thyme, chives, cloves, miso, saffron, dill, mint, nutmeg, peppermint, vanilla.

- Paprika, salt to be used with moderation

Sweets

(moderately, sugar/ sweetener free, gluten free, lactose free, milk free)

p. 153/193

Neutral: dark chocolate (without hazelnuts), rice drink, carob, carob powder, molasses, almond drink, maple syrup, white sugar, stevia, inulin.

Honey far from meals and in herbal teas or with animal proteins

Sauce/ pesto/ chutney/ paste

(you can prepare the sauce you like)

Neutral: mayonnaise (without corn starch), basil pesto (dairy and gluten free, if possible, otherwise with allowed cheese if not intolerant), green olive pesto/ sauce, jam/ marmalade with allowed fruit, parsley.

Drinks

(NO BLACK TEA)

Good: still water (room temperature), coffee, chamomile, chicory coffee, green tea.

Neutral: rice beer and millet beer (gluten free, barley free, wheat free), ginseng (with moderation), karkadè, red wine and white wine (moderately and only at lunch, it can be used to cook instead of the oil).

Herbs

Good: alfa-alfa sprouts, hawthorn, burdock, birch, chamomile, Roman chamomile, Ginseng, liquorice root, Echinacea, propolis, rosehip, dandelion, field horsetail, ginger.

Neutral: calendula, eucalyptus, peppermint, mint, hypericum, valerian, fennel seed, thyme, parsley, sage, elder.

6.5.3 People with diseases

Meat

Good: lamb, goat, rabbit, venison, rabbit, mutton.

Neutral: pheasant, turkey, liver (from beef or turkey), ostrich.

p. 154/193

Fish

Good: stone bass, pike, snails (Helix Pomatia), cod, hake, salmon, sardines, mackerel, tuna, sturgeon.

Neutral: herring, squid, caviar, carp, scallop, mussel, gilthead bream (orate), smooth-hound, perch, catfish, swordfish, cuttlefish/ squid, sole, rainbow trout, trout, goatfish, white fish.

Soya

Neutral: soya milk, tofu (gluten free), soya yoghurt

Eggs

Good: from 3 to 7 eggs per week, not fried (no butter with them).

Oils and Fats

Good: extra virgin olive oil, grape seed oil, rice oil.

Neutral: cod liver oil, linseed oil, hempseed oil.

Seeds

(walnuts and chestnuts only during autumn and winter)

Good: peanut, peanut butter, chestnuts, walnuts.

Neutral: almonds, Brazil nuts, pistachio, pine nuts, pecan nuts, macadamia nuts, hemp seeds, almond butter (to be used with moderation).

Chestnuts: do not combine them with cereals/ grains, dairy products. To be avoided during the summertime

Legumes/ beans/ pulses

You can use also beans flours (you can prepare it or use cooked beans to be mixed with eggs and other ingredient to bake bread or cake for daytime meals) – together with poultry, eggs, or fish.

Good: kidney beans, red beans, green lentils.

Neutral: cannellini beans, lentils and red lentils, peas, and green beans (you can eat these also at dinner), broad beans, yellow and green soya, mange tout, lupin beans.

Vegetables

(at least three times per day)

Good: alfa-alfa sprouts, beetroot, chard and Swiss chard, broccoli, cauliflower, cucumber, aubergine, parsnip, parsnip, sweet potatoes, celery, dandelion, parsley.

Neutral: seaweed, asparagus, carrot, Brussels sprouts, savoy cabbage, cabbage, chicory, chervil, daikon, fennel, watercress, cumin, porcini mushrooms, Bamboo sprouts, soya sprouts, endive, chestnut mushroom, green olives, lettuce (summer), leek, onion, radish, horseradish, spinach, courgette/ zucchini, ginger, truffle, pumpkin, potatoes.

Reminder:

- Garlic only if you can digest it;
- Artichoke, lettuce, spinach: to be avoided if without gallbladder;
- Onion only if you can digest it.

Juices

(same rules as per fruit) with moderation, only during summer

Good: carrot.

Spices

Good: garlic, ginger, curry, horseradish.

Neutral: bay laurel, dill, bergamot, carob, basil, cinnamon, carob, cardamom, chervil, coriander, turmeric, cumin, fennel seeds, rosemary, sage, salt, tarragon, marjoram, gluten free soya sauce, thyme, chives, cloves, miso, saffron, dill, mint, nutmeg, peppermint, vanilla.

- Paprika, salt to be used with moderation

p. 156/193

Sauce/ pesto/ chutney/ paste

(you can prepare the sauce you like)

Neutral: mayonnaise (without corn starch), basil pesto (dairy and gluten free, if possible, otherwise with allowed cheese if not intolerant), green olive pesto/ sauce, jam/ marmalade with allowed fruit, parsley.

Drinks

(NO BLACK TEA)

Good: still water (room temperature), coffee, chamomile, chicory coffee, green tea.

Neutral: rice beer and millet beer (gluten free, barley free, wheat free), ginseng (with moderation), karkadè, red wine and white wine (moderately and only at lunch, it can be used to cook instead of the oil).

Herbs

Good: alfa-alfa sprouts, hawthorn, burdock, birch, chamomile, Roman chamomile, Ginseng, liquorice root, Echinacea, propolis, rosehip, dandelion, field horsetail, ginger.

Neutral: calendula, eucalyptus, peppermint, mint, hypericum, valerian, fennel seed, thyme, parsley, sage, elder.

6.6   Unknown Blood Type

6.6.1 General

Sugary products, too much fruit, abuse of cereals (even if gluten free) can create problems to your mood, your energy level, etc. It is better to avoid dairy products (e.g., milk, cheese, cream, ice-cream, etc.). Do not mix meat and fish as this requires a lot of enzymes to be produced and dumped into the stomach by the liver and pancreas (it may cause indigestion).

It is healthier if you do not fry your food. Drink when you are thirsty.

A moderate exercise is fine (unless your GP/ Doctor suggests you not to). Practice sports that can help you to relax (e.g., yoga or Pilates) and try to rest when it is possible.

At least 30 minutes before having breakfast, get a cup (or two) of hot water with half squeezed lemon. You can also drink the hot water of the vegetables half an hour or 1 hour before your meal.

You can eat fresh vegetables as a snack together with some beans (beans only until lunch and never together with cereals or roots). You can also eat sliced cooked poultry at breakfast, lunch, snack, or dinner (but dairy free, gluten free, potato starch free, corn starch/ flour free). Dried fruit (almond, prunes) are good as snacks.

6.6.2 Healthy People

Meat

Neutral: turkey.

Fish

Good: salmon, cod, sardines, mackerel, rainbow trout, carp, stone bass, perch.

Neutral: tuna, swordfish, trout, sea bass, smooth-hound, pike, white fish.

Soya

Good: soya milk, tofu (gluten free), soya yoghurt

Eggs

Good: from 4 to 7 eggs per week, not fried (no butter with them).

Cereals and grains

(and relevant flour)

Neutral: amaranth, buckwheat (only in autumn/ winter), quinoa.

p. 158/193

Oils and Fats

Good: grape seed oil, linseed oil, extra-virgin olive oil, pumpkin seed oil, rice oil.

Neutral: sesame oil, sunflower oil, hempseed oil.

Seeds

(walnuts and chestnuts only during autumn and winter)

Good: walnuts, pumpkin seeds.

Neutral: pine nuts, almonds, chestnuts, macadamia nuts, pecan, hemp seeds, sesame seeds, sunflower seeds and butter, almond butter, walnut butter, tahini

All these kinds of butter have to be used with moderation.

Legumes/ beans/ pulses

You can use also beans flours (you can prepare it or use cooked beans to be mixed with eggs and other ingredient to bake bread or cake for daytime meals) – together with poultry, eggs, or fish.

Neutral: cannellini beans, green beans (you can eat these also at dinner), peas (you can eat these also at dinner), broad beans, mange tout, lupin bean, adzuki (red soya), black eyed beans, yellow and green soya.

Vegetables

(at least three times per day)

Good: chards, broccoli, artichokes, chicory, carrots, onion, parsnip, alfalfa sprouts, soya sprouts, parsley (fresh, not cooked), leak, spinach, turnip, dandelion, pumpkin, beet tops, squash, savoy cabbage, Jerusalem's artichoke, endive.

Neutral: seaweed, asparagus, beetroot, cauliflower, Brussels' sprouts, cucumber, cabbage, daikon, fennel, porcini, green olives, red radicchio, radish, rocket, shallot, celery, black/ white truffle, courgette.

Reminder:

- Garlic only if you can digest it;
- Artichoke, lettuce, spinach: to be avoided if without gallbladder;
- Onion only if you can digest it.

Fruit

(moderately, only at breakfast and with animal proteins or nuts)

Good: figs (fresh and dry), plums, prunes (check the label: no added sugar), apricot, pineapple, cherry, grapefruit, sultana, lemons, blackberry.

Neutral: watermelon, avocado, Sharon fruit/ persimmon, carob, dates, kiwi, raspberry, lemon (on fish), pomegranate, apple, blueberry, papaya, prickly pear, peach, pear, grapefruit, grape, gooseberry, blackcurrant, redcurrant, elder.

Jam: alone, as a snack, or with animal proteins. Jam never together with cereals/ roots/ flours.

Juices

(same rules as per fruit) with moderation, only during summer

Good: carrot.

Spices

Good: tamari sauce (gluten free), soya miso (gluten free), mustard (without vinegar), ginger.

Neutral: bay laurel, aniseed, basil, bergamot, cinnamon, coriander, cumin, turmeric, curry, fennel seeds, rosemary, sage, salt, thyme, chives, brewer's yeast, nutmeg, saffron, mint.

Sweets

(moderately, sugar/ sweetener free, gluten free, lactose free, milk free)

Neutral: carob, carob powder, soya drink, almond drink, stevia, inulin.

Honey far from meals and in herbal teas or with animal proteins

p. 160/193

Sauce/ pesto/ chutney/ paste

(you can prepare the sauce you like)

Neutral: artichoke paste, green olive paste, basil pesto (dairy and gluten free), mayo (without vinegar), jam/ marmalade with allowed fruit, parsley and soya sauce, mustard without vinegar.

Drinks

(NO BLACK TEA)

Good: still water (room temperature), chicory coffee, green tea, (with moderation, at lunch, it can be used to cook instead of the oil), vegetable water (at least half an hour before a meal).

Neutral: fennel tea, chamomile, white and red wine (moderately and only at lunch, it can be used to cook instead of the oil), soy milk (no added sugar/ sweeteners), almond milk (no added sugar/ sweetener), rice milk (no added sugar/ sweeteners).

Herbs

Good: Roman chamomile, chamomile, ginger, dandelion, rosehip, ginger, St. John's wort, propolis, valerian.

Neutral: birch, calendula, sage (not to be used if you are pregnant or breastfeeding, daytime only), hawthorn, linden, fennel seeds, raspberry, mulberry, peppermint, parsley, liquorice root (if blood pressure is not high), verbena.

6.6.3 People with diseases

Meat

Neutral: turkey.

Fish

Good: salmon, cod, sardines, mackerel, rainbow trout, carp, stone bass, perch.

Neutral: tuna, swordfish, trout, sea bass, smooth-hound, pike, white fish.

Soya

Good: soya milk, tofu (gluten free), soya yoghurt

Eggs

Good: from 4 to 7 eggs per week, not fried (no butter with them).

Oils and Fats

Good: grape seed oil, linseed oil, extra-virgin olive oil, pumpkin seed oil, rice oil.

Neutral: sesame oil, sunflower oil, hempseed oil.

Seeds

(walnuts and chestnuts only during autumn and winter)

Good: walnuts, pumpkin seeds.

Neutral: pine nuts, almonds, chestnuts, macadamia nuts, pecan, hemp seeds, sesame seeds, sunflower seeds and butter, almond butter, walnut butter, tahini.

All these kinds of butter have to be used with moderation.

Legumes/ beans/ pulses

You can use also beans flours (you can prepare it or use cooked beans to be mixed with eggs and other ingredient to bake bread or cake for daytime meals) – together with poultry, eggs, or fish.

Neutral: cannellini beans, green beans (you can eat these also at dinner), peas (you can eat these also at dinner), broad beans, mange tout, lupin bean, adzuki (red soya), black eyed beans, yellow and green soya.

Vegetables

(at least three times per day)

p. 162/193

Good: chards, broccoli, artichokes, chicory, carrots, onion, parsnip, alfalfa sprouts, soya sprouts, parsley (fresh, not cooked), leak, spinach, turnip, dandelion, pumpkin, beet tops, squash, savoy cabbage, Jerusalem's artichoke, endive.

Neutral: seaweed, asparagus, beetroot, cauliflower, Brussels' sprouts, cucumber, cabbage, daikon, fennel, porcini, green olives, red radicchio, radish, rocket, shallot, celery, black/ white truffle, courgette.

Reminder:

- Garlic only if you can digest it;
- Artichoke, lettuce, spinach: to be avoided if without gallbladder;
- Onion only if you can digest it.

Juices

(same rules as per fruit) with moderation, only during summer

Good: carrot.

Spices

Good: tamari sauce (gluten free), soya miso (gluten free), mustard (without vinegar), ginger.

Neutral: bay laurel, aniseed, basil, bergamot, cinnamon, coriander, cumin, turmeric, curry, fennel seeds, rosemary, sage, salt, thyme, chives, brewer's yeast, nutmeg, saffron, mint.

Sauce/ pesto/ chutney/ paste

(you can prepare the sauce you like)

Neutral: artichoke paste, green olive paste, basil pesto (dairy and gluten free), mayo (without vinegar), jam/ marmalade with allowed fruit, parsley and soya sauce, mustard without vinegar.

Drinks

(NO BLACK TEA)

p. 163/193

Good: still water (room temperature), chicory coffee, green tea, (with moderation, at lunch, it can be used to cook instead of the oil), vegetable water (at least half an hour before a meal).

Neutral: fennel tea, chamomile, white and red wine (moderately and only at lunch, it can be used to cook instead of the oil), soy milk (no added sugar/ sweeteners), almond milk (no added sugar/ sweetener), rice milk (no added sugar/ sweeteners).

Herbs

Good: Roman chamomile, chamomile, ginger, dandelion, rosehip, ginger, St. John's wort, propolis, valerian.

Neutral: birch, calendula, sage (not to be used if you are pregnant or breastfeeding, daytime only), hawthorn, linden, fennel seeds, raspberry, mulberry, peppermint, parsley, liquorice root (if blood pressure is not high), verbena.

7 Ancient Western Medicine Diet

In a manner similar to Tibetan medicine and other Eastern medicinal systems, the ABO-PLUS™ approach does focus on digestion and diet as the main therapy. Tibetan medicine sees every aspect of living a life as a factor to pre-dispose an individual to disease. But, digestion, being the most important factor, is the activity that can restore balance to the body. It is also the activity which can cause an imbalance in any organ or part of the body, because of issues concerning digestion (indigestion).

All other Eastern medicinal systems agree with this basic concept. By providing wrong food or impairing digestion in other ways, the energy becomes unharmonious and may disrupt the normal processes in other organs. Other misalignments may occur, and these will have to be reset/corrected by a proper diet.

ABO-PLUS™ system is based also on ancient Western tradition and takes into consideration its long-forgotten wisdom. Not long forgotten because many tricks have been just lost by one generation (our grandparents know some of these). Ancient Western medicine is based on the knowledge of Hippocrates and Galen. This knowledge was then perfected in the middle ages by Unani Tibb and St. Hildegard of Bingen. We shall then focus on these masters and their insight.

7.1 Ancient Western Tradition

The main criterion for dieting in the ancient wester medicine is the constitution of an individual. No kidding. We have talked about this for the whole book and now is the time to use it!

Let's remind ourselves of the basic constitutional structure of the four Western biotypes (see Figure 35).

Figure 35. Properties of Western Biotypes (Ancient Medicine)

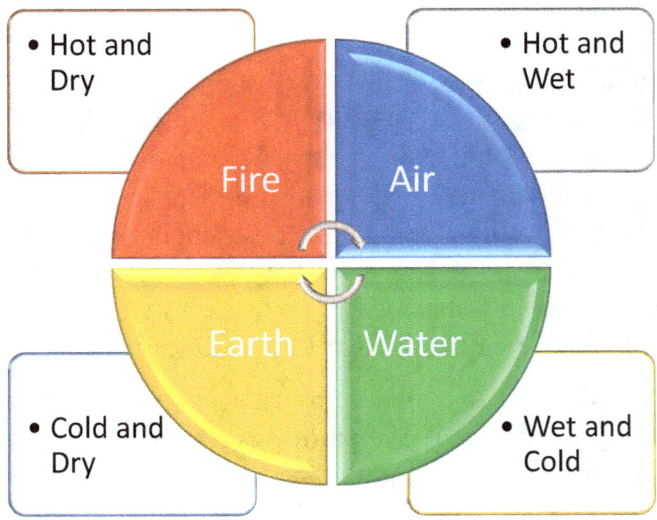

There is nothing new here in terms of qualities/properties given to each element, as the Greek and Romans intended them. All ancient western philosophers knew the basic properties of the four elements. Fire is hot (clearly) and dry, Air is hot and wet, Water is cold and wet (of course), and Earth is cold and dry. They are so simply straightforward that it is almost intuitive.

And this was reflected in the constitutional structure of the human body. As an example, one can think of a fire biotype who, being tendentially hot, can resist to cold temperatures much better than other biotypes. And indeed, it may happen that they do not "feel" (as a sensation) the cold weather as much as the other biotypes.

Hippocrates and his followers (practitioners) differentiate the diet of the healthy ("diaita hygienon", hygiene) from that of the sick. Of course, what a healthy person can "master", that is digest, may not necessarily be true for a sick individual. The reason lies in the concept of digestive energy. The human body needs to spend energy to break down foodstuff and process it. The ancient cultures knew this and thus formulated specific diets for those who were impaired. By providing easily "digestible" foods to sick patients, these would more quickly focus their energy to rebalance their disequilibrated state back to health.

In cases of acute diseases and during the crisis itself, there's mention solid food for the sick, but only dieting with gruel ("ruphemata") and hydromel as a drink.

Other secondary aspects concern the types of meals depending on the season. According to the Hippocratic knowledge, each of the four seasons is defined by two elemental qualities that affect the body. The two qualities are hot/cold and dry/wet. They are so divided: winter is cold and wet, spring hot and wet; summer hot and dry, autumn cold and dry. Hence, depending on the season you are in, one is supposed to eat food with the opposite qualities with respect to that season.

An example is the fact that in winter (being cold and wet), it is best to eat hot and dry food to counterbalance the quality of the season.

p. 167/193

7.2   Food Properties

And what is exactly considered a hot, cold, dry, or wet food? Well, the qualities of foods are loosely summarized in their external physical qualities. Some of their physical qualities are certainly clearly seen with the naked eye. For example, a wet food is best in summer while a hot food is best in winter. This is because the qualities of the food are opposite those of the season in order to moderate them.

A list of foods with specific qualities can be found in several books available in many libraries. The older they are the more consistent with ancient tradition they are. Most famous are St. Hildegard of Binge's manual (Physica). But others include writers such as:

- the book "Natura dei Cibi" of Baldassare Pisanelli, 1584;

- "Healths Improvement or Rules comprising and discovering the nature, method and manner of preparing all sorts of food", written by Thomas Muffett and corrected by Christopher Bennet in 1655;

- "A Treatise On the Nature of Aliments, or Foods, in General" of Frederick Hoffman, written in 1761.

Although old, one might think that they lack value. On the contrary, they still maintain a greater understanding of the hot and cold relationships with food than any modern treatise. Unfortunately, most of this information becomes lost the closer we get to our own time (contemporary epoch).

An incomplete list of the qualities or properties of foods is provided based on the experience and supranatural insight of St. Hildegard of Bingen.

p. 168/193

Table 13. List of Food Properties

Foods	Hot/Cold	Wet/Dry	Comment
Wheat	hot	-	Only with the entire grain
Spelt	hot	-	Easy to digest
Barley	cold	-	Problematic food
Cinnamon	hot	dry	
Curcuma	hot	-	
Nutmeg	hot	dry	
Cumin	warm	dry	
Galingale	totally hot	-	Very helpful spice
Wild thyme	hot	balanced	
Savory	hot	moist	
Sage	hot	dry	
Rue	warm	moist	
Feverfew[1]	warm	dryish	Useful for digestion
Psyllium	cold	-	
Fennel	warm	balanced	
Hemp	hot	-	Healthy
Poppy	cold	moist	
Hyssop	hot	dry	Takes out bad humors
Peas	cold	moist	A bit phlegmatic
Broad bean	hot	-	Easy to digest
Turnip	warm		Easy to digest
Plantain	hot	dry	
Licorice	warm	-	Helpful for digestion
Spearmint	hot	balanced	It warms the stomach
Salmon	cold	-	
Northern pike	warm	-	
Sea bream	warm	-	
Perch	hot	-	Healthy meat
Chicken	warm/cold	-	
Quail	hot	moist	
Deer	hasty hot	-	Healthy meat
Roe deer	hot/warm	-	Healthy meat
Bison	hot	-	Healthy meat
Lamb	warm	-	Cold in winter
Pig	hot	-	Full of mucous (not healthy)

1 = also called "Bertram"
The "-" means that it is neutral or not defined.

p. 169/193

7.3 Supplements

7.3.1 Introduction

Vitamins and minerals, collectively referred to as supplements. The term "micronutrients" is also used and is identical to supplements. Everybody should recognize the importance of micronutrients and their impact on health. Micronutrients may be divided into essential and non-essential. Essential nutrients are deemed so because their deficiency (lack) brings about a disease or illness.

The main scope of micronutrients is to do two essential things. One is to help the body transform all macronutrients (proteins, fats, and carbohydrates) obtained from food into the stuff that can be used by the body. Two is to help the body do all other normal biological processes. Essentially, they work a lot like tools, deliberately used by the human body to maintain health and fight disease.

The clinical conditions, known as deficiencies, occur when too little amounts of micronutrients are consumed. These deficiencies are commonly thought to be avoided by consuming a normal healthy and varied diet. Or even by supplementing with an adequate, internationally recognized, standardized "daily intake" (amount) of micronutrients from foods.

But is this actually true?

Without going into details, it is good to known that both the EU and the US have agreed upon the lowest daily doses of micronutrients. These lowest doses are necessary for every human being to avoid the clinical manifestation of the deficiency condition. The problem is that this minimum dose is frequently believed to be the also the correct daily dose. Indeed, this minimum dose has also been called the "recommended dietary allowance" (RDA).

7.3.2 Correct Amounts

There are several reasons why these RDA are way below the actual needed amounts for every person. One has to consider the lifespan of each individual and how many years one has taken amounts below the needed. Then by multiplying this to the lifespan, one would obtain the actual "missing amount". This is the deficiency. So, the actual optimum amount for each person may be far from the recommended quantities. And this depends on individual conditions.

Another reason is the fact that micronutrients do not work alone. They work together, they need each other to become a tool. A hammer alone would be almost worthless without the anvil. The same thing occurs for vitamins and minerals.

They are like the pieces of a puzzle that the human body must put together. This is why most often you will find full micronutrient supplementation in the market. But, to define an adequate supplementation regimen should always be done personally by considering all factors. This to avoid or reduce micronutrient deficiency.

One other reason is the presence of foodstuff that bind to and seize micronutrients. These sequester molecules simply do not allow them to be available biologically (that is absorbable and useful). We know that this is the case for many people and is a complex issue that we will not discuss further.

One other major concern is that these amounts are merely not present in foods, anymore. And why are they not there. Because they have been lost. I know, you might ask. How come?

Several explanations have been known for decades, really. But the most important is surely soil impoverishment over long periods of time. This is caused by soil acidification, erosion, and degradation with a consequential loss of nutrients.

Without investigating all the possible causes of soil impoverishment, we need to just consider its consequences.

p. 171/193

If micronutrients are deficient in soils, they would not only have an impact on crop production, but also on human and livestock nutrition and health. This aspect of micronutrient impoverishment has abundantly been studied over the past few decades. We should ask ourselves: why do veterinarians give supplements to livestock? Because farmers and veterinarians know how to correct micronutrient deficiency in vegetation and in livestock.

This is not something new. It has been known since at least the 1960s.

Several supplementation methods (vitamin–mineral pre-mixes) have been used effective to improve micronutrient nutrition for livestock and humans. Among these are biofortification of foods and the use of supplements, as the most common and familiar approaches.

And this concept is not novel.

Since supplementation has been shown to be utterly successful on animals, it seems the most sensible solution also for humans.

The only remaining point is to define daily amounts to be consumed (that is, their actual quantities). Both the EU and the US Health authorities have set the dose of the nutrients to the highest amount without any adverse events. These limits are called upper limits (ULs).

We should choose a dose of a micronutrient that can maximally be utilized by our body. Of course, everything should be discussed with your personal Medical Doctor.

A list of current ULs for vitamins and minerals from both the EU and US Authorities is presented in Table 14.

Table 14. UL and RDVs from EU and US sources (per day)

Micronutrient	EFSA 2006 (UL)	DRI 2019 (UL)	DRV 2019	RDA
Vitamin A	20 mg (n/d)	3000 µg	700 µg	770 µg
Vit. B1 (Thiamine)	n/d	n/d	0.9 mg	1.4 mg
Vit. B2 (Riboflavin) [1]	n/d	n/d	1.4 mg	1.4 mg
Vit. B3 (Niacin or Nicotinic acid)	n/d	35 mg	13 mg	18 mg
Vit. B5 (Pantothenic Acid)	n/d	n/d	n/a	6 mg
Vit. B6 (Pyridoxine) [1]	25 mg	100 mg	1.2 mg	1.9 mg
Vit. B7 (Biotin)	n/d	n/d	n/a	30 µg
Vit. B9 (Folic Acid)	1000 µg	1000 µg	300 µg	600 µg
Vit. B12 (Cobalamin)	n/d	n/d	1.5 µg	2.6 µg
Vit. C (ascorbic acid) [1]	n/d	2000 mg	50 mg	85 mg
Vit. D	100 µg	100 µg	20 µg	15 µg
Vit. E	300 mg	2000 mg	n/a	15 mg
Vit. K	n/d	n/d	n/a	90 µg
Iron	n/d	45 mg	14.8 mg	27 mg
Zinc	25 mg	40 mg	7.0 mg	11 mg
Iodine	600 µg	1100 µg	140 µg	220 µg
Magnesium (Mg)	250 mg *	350 mg	270 mg	350 mg
Manganese	n/d	11 mg	n/d	2.0 mg
Copper	n/d	10000 µg	1.2 mg	1000 µg

p. 173/193

Micronutrient	EFSA 2006 (UL)	DRI 2019 (UL)	DRV 2019	RDA
Calcium [2]	2500 mg	2500 mg	700 mg	1000 mg
Phosphorus	n/d	3.5 g/d	550 mg	700 mg
Chromium	n/d	n/d	n/a	30 µg
Boron	10 mg	20 mg	n/a	n/a
Fluoride	7 mg	10 mg	n/a	3 mg
Chloride	n/d	3.6 g	2500 mg	2.3 g
Molybdenum	0.6 mg	2000 µg	n/a	50 µg
Nickel	n/d	1.0 mg	n/a	n/a
Potassium	n/d	n/d	3500 mg	4.7 g
Selenium	300 µg	400 µg	60 µg	60 µg
Sodium	n/d	n/d	1600 mg	1.5 g/d
Tin	n/d	n/a	n/a	n/a
Vanadium	25 mg	n/d	n/a	n/a
Lipoic Acid	n/d	n/a	n/a	n/a
Fatty Acids • DHA • EPA • DPA	n/d	n/a	n/a	n/a

n/d=not defined
Definitions: DRI = Daily Recommended Intake; DRV = Daily Recommended Values; EFSA = European Food Safety Agency; RDA = Recommended Daily Allowance
Those vitamins and minerals highlighted in green represent the micronutrients which do not have a defined UL. Therefore, there is no risk in increasing the dosages per day well beyond the limits recommended by the international authorities.
Table taken from Menapace (2023).
1 = The only adverse event is stimulus to go to the bathroom.
2 = Calcium is not really a good mineral as it should be substituted with magnesium.

Whenever the ULs are unknown, it means that those micronutrients can been given to healthy and unhealthy individuals at doses of at least 100 times the RDA, without any adverse reaction. I repeat, without ANY adverse effect or event, because it is not known. The health authorities have confirmed this.

Whatever the case, some examples of no-UL micronutrients include vitamins B1, B2 and B3. No adverse events were noted (only some beneficial effects), in any experiments done thy the Health Authorities, confirming again that an UL could not be established. Similar experiments have been done for several other vitamins and minerals for over many decades confirming that no UL can be proven.

These experimental results suggest that micronutrients can be assimilated at much higher doses than normally advocated by Health Authorities (up to 50-100 times), without risks.

7.3.3 Vitamins & Minerals

A few considerations for each major micronutrient will be proposed hereafter. The scope is to show their importance and how the amounts can be calculated and retrieved in market supplements. These are the amounts necessary for maximal health maintenance.

It is best to take amounts just below the UL, where these exist.

7.3.3.1 Vitamin C

Vitamin C, ascorbic acid, is the most important vitamin of them all. That's why it is reported as first. The data on vitamin C (ascorbic acid) is vast and multitudes of studies have been completed since the 1940s. The odd thing is that vitamin C is much more than a vitamin and it resembles a macronutrient in the relative amounts that can be consumed.

The vitamin is remarkably nontoxic at high levels (10 to 100 times the RDA, when taken orally). There is no evidence suggesting that vitamin C is carcinogenic or teratogenic or that it causes adverse reproductive effects.

7.3.3.2 *Vitamin D*

Vitamin D (with chemical name calciferol, which is the D2) is unique among vitamins. The reason is that it is a substance photosynthesized in the skin through solar ultraviolet B radiation. The actual active form is Vitamin D3 (called cholecalciferol). This last one is the biologically useful form of this vitamin, but we shall continue to refer it as vitamin D.

Vitamin D has a major biologic function in humans to maintain serum calcium and phosphorus concentrations within the normal range. Although sunlight triggers the formation of Vitamin D in human skin, studies proved that there's always a high prevalence of Vitamin D deficiency. So, it is practically useless to get solar exposure. We need to supplement this with enough to supply for the general daily needs of the body. This amounts to 125 µg (microgram corresponding to 5000 IU [international units]) per day.

It regulates the metabolism of calcium. But calcium is not that good, and magnesium is better and should be used as a substitute.

7.3.3.3 *Iodine*

Iodine is the first mineral. It is actually not a mineral but an element of the periodic table. A fact very few people know is that iodine is a key micronutrient present in minute quantities in food. Too little though.

Iodine is an essential dietary element for mammals being required for the synthesis of the thyroid hormones. The only natural sources for humans and animals are the iodides in food and water. So, supplementation of 1 mg a day would be the minimal amount for the human body. We should note that Japanese people living on the coast within their food (algae) take up to 10 mg a day, normally.

p. 176/193

7.3.3.4 *Vitamin B1*

The first vitamin of the B group is Thiamine. Thiamine has many functions. Vitamin B1 is essential in energy metabolism and is used extensively by lipid (fat) and nucleotide synthesis enzymes. Thiamine is required as a coenzyme in all tissues. Its supplementation in suitable quantities may also reduce or stop neurodegenerative diseases and treat delirium. Amounts of up to 100 mg can be given without adverse events.

7.3.3.5 *Vitamin B2*

Riboflavin (Vitamin B2) is another water soluble and heat stable vitamin. This vitamin is necessary for normal human development, lactation, physical performance, and reproduction. It is used by the body to metabolize fats, protein, and carbohydrates. This vitamin is not present in sufficient quantities in vegan diets and should be supplemented regularly. Amounts of up to 100 mg can be given without adverse events.

7.3.3.6 *Vitamin B3*

Niacin is the simplest but also the most important water-soluble B complex vitamin.

Niacin is linked to energy pathways and DNA repair and replication. Amounts of up to 300 mg can be given without adverse events.

7.3.3.7 *Vitamin B5*

Pantothenic acid (vitamin B5) is a component of coenzyme A (CoA), involved in fatty acid metabolisms. This essential to life vitamin is a fundamental cofactor in a wide variety of metabolic processes. Amounts of up to 100 mg can be given without adverse events.

7.3.3.8 *Vitamin B6*

Vitamin B6 (also known as pyridoxine) is yet another water-soluble vitamin. Its importance is linked to its function as a co-enzyme in protein metabolism and in the development of the central nervous system Amounts of up to 100 mg can be given without adverse events.

7.3.3.9 *Vitamin B7*

Biotin, an essential water-soluble B-vitamin (known as cofactor, Vitamin H). It has many key roles in human metabolism, as a cofactor for enzymes involved in fatty acid synthesis and oxidation and for mitochondrial metabolism. Although biotin is widely distributed in natural food, its concentration varies substantially. For example, liver contains biotin at about 100 µg/100 g whereas fruits and most meats contain only about 1 µg/100 g. Amounts of up to 100 µg can be given without adverse events.

7.3.3.10 *Vitamin B12*

Vitamin B12, also known as cobalamin, can be present in several forms and is crucial for DNA synthesis and for cellular energy production. Amounts of up to 100 µg can be given without adverse events.

Vitamin B12 deficiency is common and is associated with gastrointestinal complaints related.

7.3.3.11 *Vitamin A*

Vitamin A (β-carotene or retinol) belongs to the category of substances known as antioxidants. Antioxidants reduce the oxidative stress of a cell. Vitamin A is important for a variety of physiologic functions including normal vision, gene expression and reproduction.

7.3.3.12 *Magnesium*

Magnesium is a mineral. It is likely to be the most important mineral. It is less famous than calcium although I would not recommend taking calcium at all. There is enough calcium in water and in food for our daily needs. But for magnesium, this is not the case. Magnesium is known to help calcium remain in the bones and to reduce cramps. The best form is when it is chelated (that is linked to an organic compound). This increases considerably the absorption. Magnesium citrate or bisglycinate are among the best known chelates for this mineral. Doses up to 400 mg are safe to take.

7.3.3.13 *Conclusions*

Overall, these functions of vitamins and minerals suggest that appropriate amounts need to be consumed to avoid problems. Many such problems can manifest slowly in time as the body becomes deficient of the essential nutrients. Only in the right amounts, can we avoid deficiencies and store enough of these to be lasting for a short while. When adequate amounts are taken, we cannot just to reduce the clinical signs of deficiencies but also the subclinical and long-term issues.

The suggestion is to search for the right supplements on the market that can match the amounts that have been suggested. It is possible to take them for a long period of time or for shorter cycles, depending on your preferences. If you feel that the supplementation is aiding your physical and mental health, then continue until you are tired.

One last thing to think about: our body has been trained to deal with essential vitamins and minerals. It knows what to do with them and how to dispose of them. Maybe this is why for most vitamins we don't find ULs?

8 General Conclusions

As we have seen, this book has explained the birth of the ABO-PLUS^{TM} method as derived from the fusion between ancient constitutional medicine and the ABO blood type diet. It is a starter manual to give you a quick but strong introduction to the potential of this approach. I cannot explain all the complexities of the therapeutic potential of ABO-PLUS^{TM} in a single book, but I have given you several tips and interesting information about your body and mind and how they are interconnected.

We, humans, are truly extremely complex beings. Here we have barely scratched the surface of the vastness of scientific know-how at the basis of alternative medicine.

We, humans, are not just composed of simple human eukaryotic cells that sometimes get infected by bugs. No! We are a well-adjusted combination of other different unicellular to pluricellular organisms. Bugs of all kinds are integrated in the holobiont. This superorganism with the combined capacity of multiple organisms (many bugs) within us. As a result, all the cells and viruses belonging to all forms of life cooperate to that equilibrium we call health. If this equilibrium is perturbed, the state that originates can be called disease. The ancient medicines (including WCM) embraced this way of reasoning and the witnesses of old sagaciously embellished their medicinal systems with this universal understanding of life for which disease has to be juxtaposed with a return to the original state of equilibrium. And all ancient medicines knew this and thus used, as main device for the correction of disharmonious states, the diet which was seen as a good method for the restoration of the equilibrium between the energies (microorganisms) in the body.

This explains very well the reasons of our difference as humans. True, the explanation is quite technical but nevertheless real. We are different because we have different bugs, with biochemical and physical variations on top of that.

Scientific and practical reasons have been given why we, as humans, inevitably react differently. And not just physiologically or biologically, as we have seen, but also psychologically. There are reasons behind all our responses. These factors have been taken into consideration in a true method to address the health concerns of people. The method is ABO-PLUS™.

For the very first time, ABO PLUS, can explain why different people obtain different results. With this method you know why you can't achieve your goals using the same strategies and diets as other people do. So, you will not be frustrated anymore, because you know how to circumvent this.

p. 181/193

And most importantly you know now how to classify yourself and based on your structure (body make or biotype) and ABO blood type, you know:

1. what to expect from yourself;
2. how to take advantage of your body's characteristics;
3. how to maximize any gain.

These two different factors, belonging to the genetics of our own human body have been put together in a simple and usable matrix. Each person has two attributes which make us biochemically and physically different from others. But within these bounds we can truly define ourselves and resolve most issues.

No one single physician or scientist has or ever will know everything that there is to know about medicine or science. Not even any theory alone can entertain completely the whole medicinal or scientific knowledge base. We can get close but never get there. Notwithstanding this, ABO-PLUS™ has come close by putting together two successful traditions.

And this is exactly what we have tried to do here.

Only through an exhaustive and well-balanced integration of the various medicines can we understand health and righteously foster it.

The bottom line is that adapting these forms of biotypology ABO-PLUS™ can offer:

1. a cheaper or more problem-free integrative (or alternative, based on your case) practice to conventional therapeutic routines in managing chronic diseases; and

2. a more reliable remedy with fewer side effects than some modern therapies (when possible).

This is a win-win situation, especially in the western Countries, both for the physicians (who can increase the supply of very effective and more painless therapies) and the patients.

p. 182/193

The distinctive experience (of each individual) compels us to continue to strive to treat every human as a unique and special person.

ABO-PLUS™ is the fusion of the ABO blood type diet and the Western form of ancient medicine. It has been blended into a matrix, a truly holistic and personalized medical system that everybody can learn.

More recently a new medicinal system, the ABO blood type diet was established. This diet or system has taken a stronger place in the scientific arena through the experimental confirmation of its main mechanism of action by fields related to the glycoscience (especially glycobiology). Inevitably, microscopic bugs (bacteria), fungi and other unicellular organisms have been shown to feed off on glycans which are both produced (ABO and others) and absorbed (diet) by the human body and the suitable balance of diet will interfere in this cycle. Time has come to secure all these advances in knowledge from ancient and modern medicine and combine them into a new medicinal system, ABO PLUS™. ABO PLUS™, that is the ABO-WCM biotypology, can factually better explain the reality of the holobiont and completely transform modern science into a truly personalized approach.

The healing interventions heralded by ABO PLUS™ is based on nutritional (i.e., what they should tendentially eat and drink) and physical therapies depending on their constitution with the use of natural (vitamins and minerals) and herbal products.

To conclude, ABO PLUS™ recognizes that we all are similar (as human beings) but also different in ways that can be properly defined (with known characteristics). ABO PLUS™ accepts these differences and similarities in a novel defined classification system. ABO PLUS™ system of classification will allow practitioners and patients to better appreciate each individual physical and physiological distinctiveness. ABO PLUS™ can uncover most if not all of our limits and potentialities as they belong to our bodies. Moreover, once known, we can use this knowledge to our benefit

p. 183/193

by choosing the remedies most suitable for each person (personalized and customized therapies).

The hope is that in the future, people will improve on this system to propose to people an always superior and better chance to understand and resolve all heath issues.

9 Appendix

9.1 List of Tables

9.2 List of Figures

p. 187/193

10 Essential Bibliography

Since this is not a study (technical) book, all manuscripts are not reported except for the essential. For a detailed bibliography please see the references in bold (two books), where all references are present.

1. Duvernier 1965. Etude des causes de l'échec scolaire en fin de cycle d'observation chez les enfants bien doués. In: Enfance, tome 18, n°1-3. Les conditions de vie et de travail de l'écolier Enseignements élémentaire, secondaire, technique. pp. 393-410.
2. Emtiazy, M., Keshavarz, M., Khodadoost, M., Kamalinejad, M., Gooshahgir, S. A., Bajestani, H. S., & Alizad, M. (2012). Relation between body humors and hypercholesterolemia: An Iranian traditional medicine perspective based on the teaching of Avicenna. Iranian Red Crescent Medical Journal, 14(3), 133.
3. Hildegard S, Berger M. 1999. On natural philosophy and medicine: selections from Cause et cure. DS Brewer
4. Hildegard S., 1998. Physica. The Complete English Translation of Her Classic Work on Health and Healing. Translated from Latin by Priscilla Throop.
5. Kim, J.Y., Pham, D.D. and Koh, B.H., 2011. Comparison of Sasang constitutional medicine, traditional Chinese medicine and Ayurveda. Evidence-Based Complementary and Alternative Medicine, 2011.
6. Levy JD. 2011. Curing the Incurable. Vitamin C, Infectious Diseases, and Toxins. Fourth Edition. MedFox Publishing LLC, Henderson, NV (US)
7. Little, J.M., 2014. The Homoeopathic Compendium by David Little. Dharamsala, IN: Omnibus Global, Friends of Health.

8. Menapace, M., 2018. Recent advances in nutritional sciences: An overview of glycans and miRNAs. J Nutr Food Sci, 8, p.734.

9. Menapace, M. 2019a. The rise of the holobiont and the return of ancient medicines. *International Journal of Medical and Health Research*, 5(7); P. 38-45.

10. Menapace M. 2019b. Western Constitutional Medicine: A Primer. *International Journal of Recent Scientific Research Vol. 10, Issue, 09(D), pp. 34733-34740.*

11. Menapace M. 2019c. ABO Blood Type-Food Relationship: The Mechanism of Interaction between Food and Human Glycans. *Acta Scientific Nutritional Health.*; 3(3):03-22.

12. Menapace, M. 2020a. ABO and WCM biotypology: The secret of the holobiont. *International Journal of Molecular Biology and Biochemistry*, 2(1); P. 18-29

13. Menapace, M., 2020b. At the Edge of Alternative Medicine: the ABO-WCM System. *Journal of Medical and Clinical Sciences.* 6(01):75-85

14. Menapace, M., 2020c. Micronutrients: Joining the dots for a holobiont nutrition. *International Journal of Food Science and Nutrition.* 6(5); 21-29

15. ***Menapace, M. 2021. ABO Blood Type Diet. Biochemical Mechanisms In Molecular Nutrition. Independently Published by Amazon. ASIN: B09CGFWS7C. ISBN-13: 979-8456671066.***

16. ***Menapace, M. 2023. ABO-PLUS. The Apex of Nutrition. Independently Published by Amazon. ASIN: B0BSJ6FVPF. ISBN-13: 979-8374381894.***

17. Mozzi, P. 2012. La dieta del dottor Mozzi. 5th Ed. Piacenza, IT: Litoquick Srl

18. Oberhammer, S., 2017. Guarigione naturale con I 4 biotipi Oberhammer. Milan, IT: Mondadori.

19. Rajgurav, A., & Aphale, P. Study Of Various Constitutions With The Help Of Clarke's And Murphy's Repertory. constitution, 12(13), 14.

20. Ramos-Jiménez, A., Chávez-Herrera, R., Castro-Sosa, A. S., Pérez-Hernández, L. C., Hernández-Torres, R. P., & Olivas-Dávila, D. (2016). Body shape, image, and composition as predictors of athlete's performance. Fitness Medicine, 1(2), 19-36.

21. Sellerio, eds. 2015. Cause e Cure delle infermità. 2nd ed. Palermo, IT: Sellerio editore.

22. Senior, J.R., 2008. What is idiosyncratic hepatotoxicity? What is it not?. Hepatology, 47(6), pp.1813-1815.

23. Stern, A.M., 2016. Eugenics in Latin America. In Oxford research encyclopedia of Latin American history.